GW01163954

HOME
DOCTOR

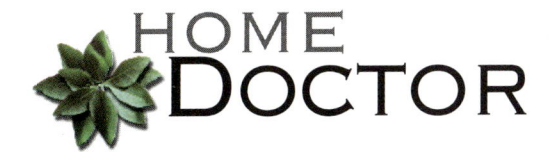

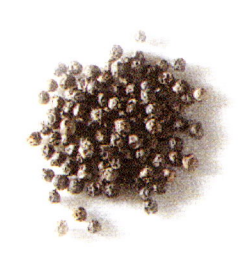

*To
Vimal Phadke
my mother-in-law
and
Pritam Sidhu
my mother
who still hold the torch alight
despite the winds of change.
It is just their way of life.*

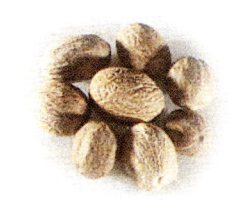

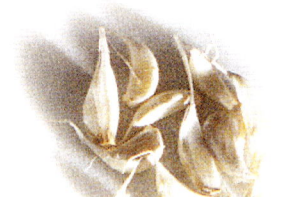

All rights are reserved. No part of this publication
may be transmitted or reproduced in any form
or by any means without the prior permission
of the publisher.

ISBN: 81-7436-167-7

Text:
Dr P. S. Phadke

Illustrations:
The Wellcome Library, London

Published by
© **Roli Books Pvt. Ltd. 2001**
Lustre Press Pvt. Ltd.
M-75 Greater Kailash, Part-II (Market)
New Delhi 110 048, India.
Phone: 6442271, 6462782
Fax: 6467185
E-mail: roli@vsnl.com
Website: rolibooks.com

Conceived and designed
at Roli CAD Centre

Printed and bound at Singapore

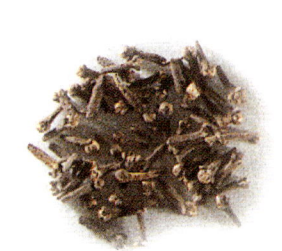

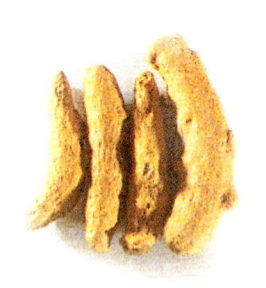

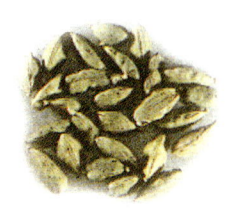

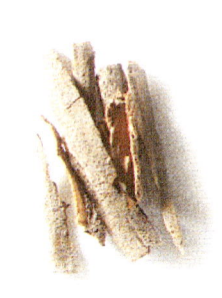

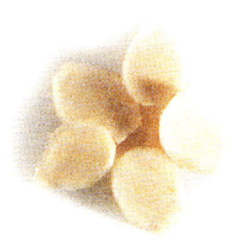

HOME DOCTOR

Dr P. S. Phadke

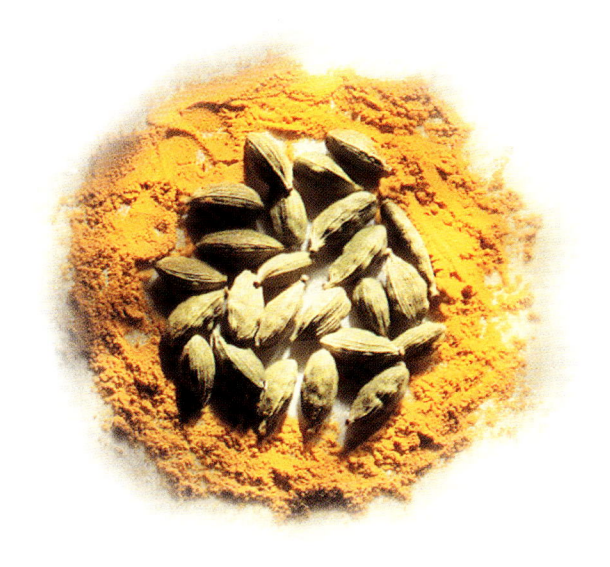

*Natural Healing Herbs,
Condiments and Spices*

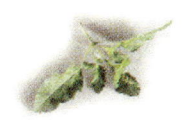

**Lustre Press
Roli Books**

ACKNOWLEDGEMENTS

○ To my mother-in-law, Vimal Phadke, for passing on to me her rich herbal heritage, which was an accepted way of life for her. Also to my mother, who put right day-to-day health problems with remedies from the kitchen or kitchen garden. As a young doctor I scoffed at their beliefs and practices, but over the years I realised that their remedies worked in a subtle, holistic manner, with no side effects—unlike allopathic medicines.

○ To Dr Narayan Balkrishan Deo, a leading allopath in Ujjain in Madhya Pradesh, India. He introduced me to the concept of holistic health care, twenty-five years ago, long before it became a fashionable term.

○ To Dr Ram Gopal of the Defence Laboratories in Jodhpur in Rajasthan, India. His work on the flora and fauna of the desert and about some of the customs of Hindu women inspired me.

○ To Ms Anuradha Singh, a scientist at the National Institute of Science, Technology and Development, Pusa Institute, Delhi, who is also a founder member of Lok Swasthya Parampara Samvardhan Samiti in Coimbatore, India. Also to FRLHT—a foundation for the revitalisation of local health traditions—in Bangalore.

○ To the writers who contributed to the compilation of the *Wealth of India* series, the *Medicinal Plants of India* volumes, and my ready reckoner, the abridged *Useful Plants of India*—a gift from Padma Shree Mr AM Gokhale.

○ To Dr (Miss) Jagdish Grover, MD, Assistant Professor in the department of pharmacology at the All India Institute of Medical Sciences, New Delhi. She has been a source of support and helped me access books on pharmacology, which provided me with the latest relevant information.

○ To Dr Kimberley Chawla, MD, for her generous sharing of thoughts and literature on alternative and complementary medicine.

○ To the Heart Care Foundation of India, where I was an assistant editor and medical journalist in the early nineties for *MEDINEWS,* and the *Indian Journal of Clinical Practice*. The Heart Care Foundation of India was founded by the late Dr (Col.) KL Chopra, a cardiologist at the Mool Chand Hospital in New Delhi. The present Chairman is the well-known Dr Deepak Chopra, the new age guru of alternative and complementary medicine in the USA.

○ To the Indian Air Force, for my husband's postings across the length and breadth of India. It gave me the opportunity of interacting with the wives and female relatives of Air Force personnel, who provided me with a treasure trove of information regarding home remedies.

○ To the team at Roli Books, for their support and cooperation.

CONTENTS

Introduction	7
How to use the book	13
Preparation of remedies	15
Fever	23
Pain	33
Head-related problems	35
General Ailments	41
Disorders of the eyes	63
Disorders of the nose	73
Mouth problems	79
Throat problems	89
Ear problems	101
Chest problems	105
Abdominal disorders	115
Urinary complaints	155
Disorders of the musculo-skeletal system	165
Skin problems	179
Stress-related disorders	233
Sexual debility and weakness	237
Gynaecological problems	241
Ailments and remedies at a glance	250
Glossary	255

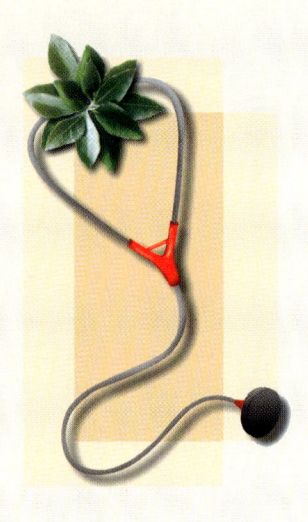

Our ancestors lived healthy, active lives depending on nature to sustain them in every way. Today we seem to have come full circle. With ailments galore and disease rampant, once again people are turning to the rich reservoir of natural resources that is our heritage.

■ INTRODUCTION

The year was 1965, and we were freshers; third year students just being introduced to clinical medicine in the outpatient department of the Lady Hardinge Medical College and Hospital for Women at New Delhi. Going through the prescribed format of complaints, history-taking, physical examination, laboratory reports and provisional diagnosis, etc., followed by a temporary prescription of say, SOS, a tablet of Paracetamol or Digene, as the case may be; till the senior registrar discussed the findings and told us what to write as the required treatment. When it came to writing a standard prescription, we were invariably asked, 'Doctor, what should I eat? Can I have cold water? Is tea harmful for me? Is this tablet to be taken with food or without? Can I have a cold water bath or not?' And I found that very often, unless it was absolutely contraindicated, we said, 'Oh, it doesn't matter, take the tablet and you will be fine.' If any complementary home remedy was suggested, we scoffed at the idea as being primitive with no meaning or bearing on the problem. Today, after over thirty years of interacting with people, I realise that there is so much in our herbal heritage, and in folklore medicine, passed down by word of mouth by women who tend the house and hearth, that tapping this treasure is an absolute necessity. Sadly, our generation of women, and those after us, who have opted for nuclear families, have lost out on this. We did not have our mothers or grandmothers close at hand to administer harmless home remedies when minor health problems arose. One only went to the doctor when a health problem began to interfere with smooth day-to-day work. Failure to notice and recognise the early symptoms when an illness begins is the main reason why it takes root and becomes difficult to treat because of its severity and stubbornness. 'It didn't bother me till now' is the real problem.

It is ironic that our herbal heritage, our folk knowledge, used by people for ages, is of negligible value today, and is scoffed at by most people if it is not available in fancy-coloured coated pills in foil strip-packing. Recent global trade conferences and treaties tend to justify this. The custodians of this herbal wealth are persuaded to supply their herbal forest produce to industry at the cost of environmental degradation, in exchange for money to buy food and consumer goods. There is no replenishing of resources, and these people, when they fall ill, turn to allopaths who prescribe the same strip-packed knowledge, which they buy back at exorbitant prices at the cost of their daily sustenance, in order to benefit industry. Modern medicine is mostly drug-dependent, and often involves invasive intervention, which is not really the answer, particularly when there is readily available, easily affordable, practical health care for all. Long before a disease is diagnosed, there are always warning signs and symptoms which can often be successfully treated with home remedies and a lifestyle change. Cures with natural remedies and lifestyle changes have the potential of reversing illness, even some very old and chronic ones. Our body has an in-built and innate ability to heal, and this should be tapped, as nature, the creator, wanted it to be. If the problem is not resolved within two to three days, or recurs after some time, a visit to the doctor is essential. This is because the doctor is professionally qualified and is in a position to correlate complaints with signs and symptoms, and after a proper physical examination, reach a tentative diagnosis, confirmed by laboratory studies, or in some cases, specialised newer diagnostic techniques—to prescribe a specific treatment modality.

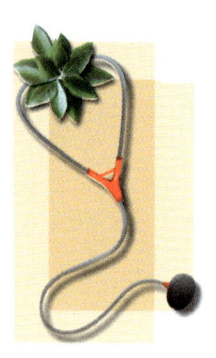

Unfortunately, treatment of disease is today a thriving industry, and it feeds obscene amounts in profits and commissions to doctors, druggists and diagnostics. Aggressive advertising and medical literature ensure that pharmaceuticals rule the roost. Maintaining the infrastructure of the health care industry takes up more money than the actual services delivered. However, a slowly increasing number of modern medicine practitioners do not rely on drugs alone. They prescribe complementary dietary and lifestyle changes, as drugs by themselves can cause various side effects, which produce 'newer' diseases. Rising

LONG BEFORE A DISEASE IS DIAGNOSED, THERE ARE ALWAYS WARNING SIGNS AND SYMPTOMS WHICH CAN OFTEN BE SUCCESSFULLY TREATED WITH HOME REMEDIES AND A LIFESTYLE CHANGE.

> CURES WITH NATURAL REMEDIES AND LIFESTYLE
> CHANGES HAVE THE POTENTIAL OF REVERSING
> ILLNESS, EVEN SOME VERY OLD AND CHRONIC ONES.

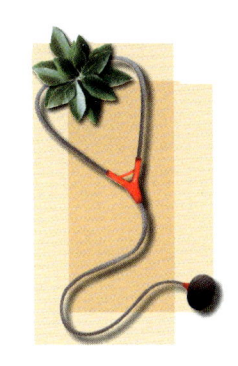

levels of literacy, health-related advocacy or awareness generated by the media, plus exorbitant drug pricing, is making the lay person or the consumer turn to more easily available, less toxic avenues of health care. This has also led to the revival of indigenous health care practices—the leading and better known ones being ayurveda, Unani, siddha, homeopathy, acupuncture, acupressure, Chinese medicine, massage, aromatherapy, meditation, yoga, reiki and pranic healing.

So we come full circle, and the woman at home is often the first to deal with headaches and 'heartaches', indigestion and insomnia; not to forget cuts and burns, nappy rashes, and much more. To aid this woman, and keeping in mind what every home has, either on the kitchen shelf or in the kitchen garden, or in and around the house, this is a comprehensive compilation of safe, time-tested in-house prescriptions to help tide over day-to-day common health complaints. Your doctor, of course, is the best person to consult should you still not feel better. Some of these remedies are complementary to allopathic treatment. Should you decide to take some of these as a complementary adjuvant to a specific prescription for a chronic disorder, e.g., diabetes, your blood-sugar levels will need to be monitored for a review of your prescription, as allopathic drug requirements may become much less.

For a health disorder to occur there has to be an agent, a host and an environment. An 'agent' is the causative factor. It may be a virus or a bacterium which causes the infection, or it may be from elements in the environment, such as fire, heat, snow, or severe cold, which may cause burns, heat stroke or frost bite; or it may just be constant nagging worries, however inconsequential, which cause cumulative stress. This leads to stress-related disorders, ranging from simple mild anxiety to violent anger, psychosis, neurosis or disorders such as hypertension, diabetes, or even cancer. The 'host' is the individual who 'catches' the infection, gets burnt, or falls prey to depression. The 'environment' is the substrate, which is largely responsible for a person being vulnerable to diseases. A weak, malnourished person will 'catch' an infection easily, as compared to a healthy, robust individual. If one is wearing an inflammable nylon dress while working next to an open flame, there is the inherent risk of getting burnt. Worrying about day-to-day affairs which are not in one's control leads to depression, just as living in the the fast lane of life leads to early burnout. All these are preventable, and to some extent fully curable if tackled in time. It must be remembered that material objects per se never cause disease. They are merely agents waiting to cause symptoms in susceptible hosts. Internal factors determine the nature of our relationship with them. Susceptibility may involve physical and chemical changes in body tissues, but those changes are initiated at another subtle realm in certain areas of the brain, which at times border on the abstract.

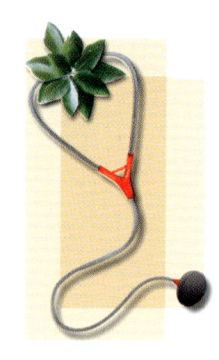

This book is an effort to make you aware of the various factors involved which cause disease, and how to arrest it in its nascent form, right at the beginning. These remedies cannot treat genetic disorders, though palliation of symptoms may be possible. Similarly, environmental or occupational health hazards or disorders are beyond the scope of this book.

Lastly, I wish to warn you about the host of so-called medical literature floating about written by people without even a basic knowledge of the medical sciences. Often remedies are suggested which are inimical to a treatment modality a person is already undergoing. Sometimes a natural remedy may be downright hazardous for a person's constitution, e.g., banana is an excellent food for maintaining good health, but is bad for a person with kidney disorder, as are ripe, sweet mangoes for a diabetic. Garlic is a much-touted remedy for anything from curing colds to coronary artery disease. The fact remains that garlic is not tolerated by all constitutions in amounts needed to cure an established disease. Chyavanprash is

> LEARNING TO BREATHE PROPERLY AND BEING AWARE OF HOW WE BREATHE IS THE SIMPLEST, SAFEST, MOST EFFECTIVE AND INEXPENSIVE WAY TO REMAIN HEALTHY IN MIND AND BODY.

an ayurvedic herbal energy /dietary supplement rich in vitamins, trace elements and natural sugars. A very weak constitution, however, may not be able to tolerate the dosage prescribed on the package literature—too much may overload and depress an already weak digestive system. Many people, particularly those with health fads, have a tendency to overdo things in a hurry to get well. This defeats the very purpose of treatment. Much confusion is also caused in the minds of people when the health sections in newspapers give conflicting reports—one day milk is good for you, and the next day it is supposed to be akin to poison; one study states that only breast milk is the best food for babies till six months of age, and the next says it is not so, that supplements are needed from three months onwards. Do not blindly follow these reports. Generations have led healthy lives on traditional diets and remedies. These have stood the test of time, whereas within the last fifty years, many treatment modalities in modern medicine have taken a 180-degree turn.

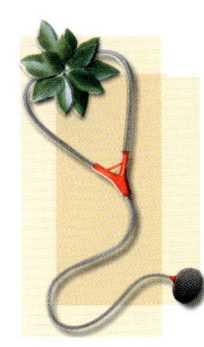

This book aims to help you learn to treat yourself by drawing from the rich reservoir of natural resources, whenever needed, and live happily in harmony with nature. Speaking of nature—God has gifted us our life-force, i.e., *prana* or life breath. Breathing is the most mysterious yet vital function of life. We live because we breathe. Breathing is the only function in the body that is totally involuntary, and yet can be fully voluntary. Learning to breathe properly and being aware of how we breathe is the simplest, safest, most effective and inexpensive way to remain healthy in mind and body. Whereas breathing is invisible, the blood in our bodies is visible, and it is vital for sustaining health and healing. Blood carries nourishment and energy to every part of the body. Hence, ensuring an adequate blood supply, i.e., maintaining the efficient circulation of blood in the body is the master key to health and healing.

Nature is mother bountiful in her healing resources. The scope of this book, however, is limited to its being a ready reckoner at home, and the remedies suggested are mainly made from condiments, spices and herbs you are most likely to have on your kitchen shelf, larder or kitchen garden. Some common flowers, shrubs and trees have also been included. Wherever diet is mentioned, the accent is on a vegetarian combination of foods. The nomenclature is one that is in common usage.

HOW TO USE THE BOOK

This book first elaborates on the causes and symptoms of ailments, then gives directions about how to prepare the remedies; after that is an explanation about how these remedies work. Next there is information given regarding what are acute problems and what are chronic conditions. The main chapters begin with two common prodromal clinical presentations of most problems—fever and pain. In the rest of the book, the body is divided into various anatomical areas, starting from the head downwords, and the symptoms presenting in that area are dealt with, even though the underlying problem may lie elsewhere. However, it is clearly indicated when one should seek specialised medical care immediately. The body's inherent capacity to heal, its mysterious ways of coping with day-to-day variations in physiological processes, in response to external or internal stimuli, and to help balance a disturbed agent host and environment equation, is the task of these remedies. However, if the ailment does not right itself within two or three days, investigations and professional intervention is needed, as these symptoms may well be the 'call attention' manifestation of a serious underlying disease. Once the actual disorder is diagnosed, and active drug treatment is started, some of these remedies may complement and enhance orthodox therapy.

Complementary remedies, which can be safely taken with established life-long drug regimens for chronic diseases, have also been given while dealing with a complaint most common to the condition, e.g., headache in relation to hypertension. These are in no way inimical. If they do not help they will not harm. They are an inherent part of our daily diets. Sometimes food combinations are such that the action of one negates the good effect of the other, and the body is unable to assimilate what it needs in order to prevent a disorder.

Note: *These remedies should only be tried for a three-day period. If there is no relief from symptoms within that time, expert opinion is needed, with specific treatment under medical supervision. The remedies can still be taken as complementary adjuvants, but with the consent of the specialist. Sometimes there are individual idiosyncrasies, depending on physical constitutional variations that need to be borne in mind. People may not be aware of this. If something does not agree with you, seek advice. The bitter taste of a remedy will remain bitter, no matter how much you sugar coat it. But something which causes you to vomit, or break into a rash, when it should not, means your body is telling you its not good for you—seek medical advice immediately. Also remember that anything taken in excess causes toxicity.*

Spices and condiments should be sun-dried and stored in airtight glass or inert containers—if you live in a place where the climate is damp, do check these periodically for fungus, mildew or small parasites which may attack them. Herbs should always be gathered fresh, early in the morning when their natural oils are at the maximum—herbal natural oils are highly volatile, and the steadily increasing heat of the ascending sun depletes them. If possible, make your own herb corner with potted herbs nurtured in pollution-free, pesticide-free and inorganic fertiliser-free soil. Use organic fertilisers only. When using dried herbs, only take half the amount you would for fresh herbs, as the active ingredient in dried herbs is more concentrated. Herbs are dried in the shade or under direct sunlight, depending on how delicate they are and how volatile their essential oils are (wherever relevant this has been specified). When boiling ingredients to prepare a remedy, use Teflon-coated, steel or heat-proof glass containers. Use a porcelain pestle and mortar to powder them or make a paste. As far as possible, make fresh prescriptions—they are the most efficacious. However, at times they may need to be stored. Store dry preparations in a cool, dark, damp-free place, and pastes or creams in the refrigerator.

■ PREPARATION OF REMEDIES

All the remedies suggested in this book are safe and easy to prepare. Try only one remedy at a time and do not mix or innovate. Some of the ingredients may be available and some may not be. Use what is easily available and what the patient is willing to take. The source of the remedies is folk knowledge, which is integral to the day-to-day life of rural people all over India, wherever modern health-care facilities are not available. However, their medical efficacy has been verified from the following publications:

- The Useful Plants of India, Publications and Information Directorate, CSIR
- Medicinal Plants of India, ICMR
- Wealth of India, CSIR
- Nutritive Value of Indian Foods, ICMR

The dosages have been the same over generations, which makes them absolutely safe. Practically all of them have been the focus of funded studies from time to time.

Herbal Teas

Add a teaspoon of dried herb or two teaspoons of fresh crushed herb to two cups of water. Bring to a boil; let it steep for 10-15 minutes. A herbal tea can be had hot or cold, unless specified in particular. Keep the vessel covered with a close-fitting lid, so that nothing is lost by way of evaporation. Most of the active ingredients or medicaments are volatile. Just bringing the concoction to a boil and steeping ensures that though volatile elements are released, they are passed into the water and remain in it. Herbal tea is sipped and rolled in the mouth for a while before it is swallowed, because the inner mucosal lining of the mouth is richly supplied with blood vessels, and the volatile oils, trace elements and vitamins in their molecular state get quickly absorbed.

Infusions

Place specified amounts of freshly-crushed herbs or coarsely pounded condiments or spices in a container, and pour a specified proportionate quantity of boiling water on them. Cover with a lid, let it cool to room temperature, then use it. Infusions can also be used as herbal teas and for inhalations.

Decoctions

These are usually prepared from the dried bark of trees, their seeds and roots—hard substances which need prolonged boiling to release their active principles. If fresh, soft plant parts are used, they need gentle handling—if at all a decoction is needed, boil it for just 3-4 minutes. The amount of raw material used is about half a cup of coarsely pounded bark/seeds/roots or crushed flowers/soft leaves/stems. To this add two cups of water and boil till only one-fourth remains. Next, strain through a soft, clean, freshly-washed, sun-dried cloth or filter, and use as recommended.

Cold Extracts

In the case of delicate plants and herbs such as rose, jasmine, marigold, hibiscus, coriander, etc., whose oils evaporate very fast, the ingredients are soaked in cold water and left 10-12 hours, or even overnight. Half a cup of raw material to a cup of water is the measure to be used.

Juices

Juices can be extracted by using an electric or hand-operated juice extractor. In the absence of these, herbs can be ground in a pestle and mortar, with a little water added to it. Then the mixture should be strained through a muslin cloth. Normally juice is extracted from Indian gooseberry, garlic, ginger, holy basil, neem, lime, onion, and many other vegetables and fruits. Juice should always be consumed fresh, immediately after extraction. Avoid storing any juice even in the refrigerator, as it tends to ferment. Stored juices also lose their vitamin content.

Powders

Powders can be made by grinding

dried ingredients in a pestle and mortar or in an electric grinder. They should be stored in clean, dry, airtight containers.

Pastes

Freshly crushed herbs or a measured quantity of spice or condiments are ground to a paste with water, milk or a particular oil, and used as suggested.

HOW THESE REMEDIES WORK

Herbs, spices, condiments, fruits and vegetables are naturally occurring gifts of nature. They have been endowed with the unique capacity to absorb inorganic substances from the earth, water, fire, air, ether, and convert them into life-giving, life-supporting vital ingredients. The human body too is a living entity, and each individual body has its own life-force which sustains it. When we look for remedies in natural substances, we want something which is easily assimilable.

The medicament present in these remedies is in the form of alkaloids, essential oils, enzymes, trace elements and minerals. Once absorbed they are assimilated only in the quantity needed by the body. The active ingredient is in the natural form needed to bind to a receptor site where the vital action has to take place, in order to balance the disturbed agent, host and environment equation. There are no synthetic constituents added, as in commercial preparations, which work on the principle that a vehicle (synthetic constituent) is needed to ensure the absorption of an arbitrarily decided, fixed amount of a drug. Modern medicine laboratory/ clinical drug trials, blind and double-blind studies, determine that a certain level of the drug has to be maintained in the body to rid it of nocuous symptoms. This by itself may initially have a beneficial effect, but sustaining pre-determined, 'scientifically' approved levels in the long run also gives rise to excess intake, drug-induced/drug dependent diseases. So the right natural

■ DOSAGE

WHATEVER IS PRESCRIBED FOR AN ADULT, HALF THAT FOR A CHILD OF 6-12 YEARS; HALF THAT FOR ONE OF 2-6 YEARS; AND HALF THAT FOR ONE 1-2 YEARS OLD. GIVE IT IN DROP DOSES TO HALF A TEASPOON TO A BABY. THE REMEDIES ARE USUALLY ADMINISTERED THREE TO FOUR TIMES A DAY.

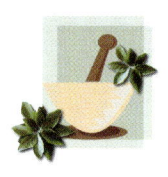

herbal remedy, taken at the first physical symptoms, manifestations or signs of disorder, helps the body's own healing mechanism. Since these are natural remedies and a part of one's daily diet, excess of any kind is excreted.

Absorption of an active principle can take place through the nasal mucosa—as in the inhalation of essential oils via inhalation from infusions. These oils may have a beneficial psychological effect—in that they relax or stimulate the mind, causing a sense of well-being, and relieving anxiety and depression. Some of these oils have antiseptic or anti-inflammatory properties. Absorption can also take place via the lining of the digestive tract—as when sipping a decoction, drinking herbal tea, or taking a herbal enema. Each active ingredient has a specific action, which is explained in the prescription, e. g., an ulcer in the mouth has a swollen base which is red and inflamed. When a herbal mouthwash is used, or a specific paste applied to the ulcer, it acts as an astringent, drawing the excess moisture out, and thereby decreasing the swelling or collection of water in the tissues. The pain of the ulcer is due to the nerve fibres in the mucosal lining responding to the stretch caused by the swelling. The sensations of pain, touch, stretch and temperature are carried by the same type of nerve fibres, and the physical response is the same—one of pain and discomfort.

Absorption of the active principle also takes place when a liniment is applied on a painful skin surface, as in a headache—irrespective of the cause of the headache—and there is a feeling of relief. This happens because the bitter/sharp ingredients in the liniment act as a counter-irritant to the pain stimulus. They block the pain receptors, so there is a sense of relief. The cause of the headache still needs to be addressed and specific action taken.

Poultices

A poultice is the application of a herbal medicament made into a warm pulpy mass and placed between two layers of warm, wet cloth. It provides moist heat. The active principle seeps through the damp cloth, soothing the area. In the case of a boil, it draws impurities and fluid out. Often it causes a boil to burst, thus bringing relief. This normally occurs within a few hours. Sometimes a fresh poultice has to be applied every few hours. However, it should not be applied for more than 12-14 hours, as it may cause local irritation.

In some remedies, massage is

suggested with the application of a particular oil. The physical action of massaging increases the circulation in the area. Better circulation means that more blood rushes to the site. More blood means more oxygen, the life-force of any living cell. This ensures that energised, prompt healing begins, and the debris of tissue damage/ metabolic waste products are hastily removed by the white blood cells, which are the first line of defence. The debris or waste products are either engulfed and destroyed or excreted.

Massaging a specific area gives physical comfort because it relieves the tenseness and the pain caused by the stretching of the skin. Mental tension or physical stress/stretching unwittingly knots the muscles in a state of sustained spasm, which a gentle, firm massage relieves. Mental stress and tension affect the immune system in a negative way, and resistance to disease is lowered. Massage also includes the unexplained, yet vital emotional advantage of touch. Psychiatric and psychological studies have proved that touch is a healing medium—an essential part of tender loving care (TLC), so important for quick recovery. The mind-body relationship is

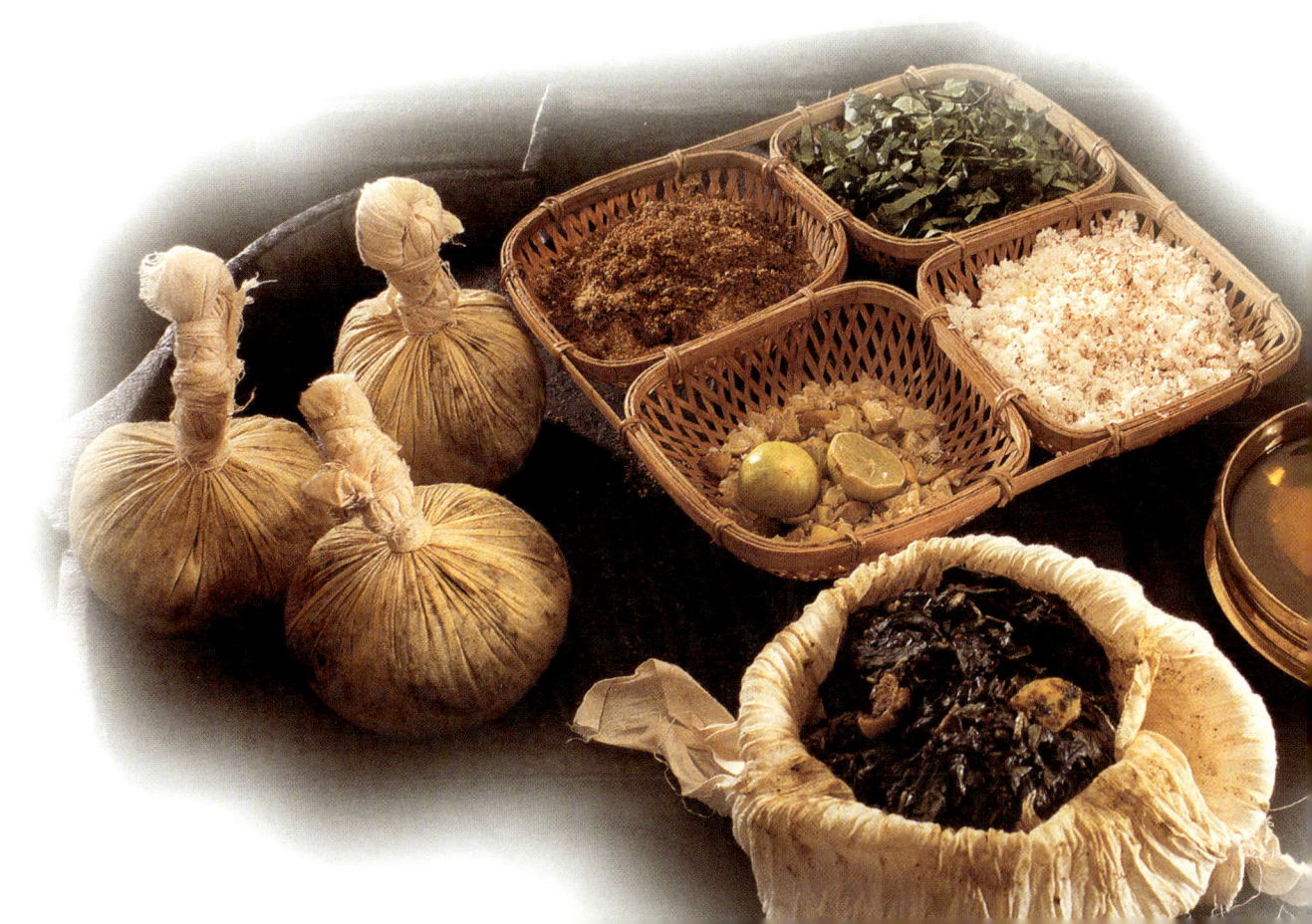

What is meant by acute and chronic illness

An acute disease or disorder is one which occurs suddenly, or at short notice, the total duration of the illness being short, the intensity of discomfort being more, and it may or may not be self-limiting in nature, e. g., infections such as common colds, chicken pox, measles, mumps, etc. A head injury, heart attack, stroke and rapidly progressing cancers are all acute conditions.

A chronic illness is a slowly progressing disease or disorder, which may respond to continuous treatment or it may not—the symptoms go through phases of remission or exacerbation. With active treatment the progression may be temporarily halted. However, the condition is rarely fully treated. With monitored maintenance therapy, a certain amount of relief is possible, and the person can live a fairly comfortable life, compatible with societal requirements. Untreated, the illness lingers, leading to debility, disability, and finally, a totally preventable early demise.

A chronic illness may be the result of an inadequately treated acute illness, e.g., repeated chest infections leading to chronic bronchitis, or it may be a degenerative disorder such as hypertension, a metabolic condition such as diabetes, or an auto-immune one like rheumatoid arthritis.

Sometimes acute episodes occur in the progression of a chronic illness. These are called acute chronic phases, e. g., an acute attack of arthritic pain in an established case of rheumatoid arthritis—there are acute phases and remissions. Similar phases also occur in the progression of asthma, hypertension, diabetes and cancer.

Acute cases need timely and active professional medical treatment. Chronic cases can benefit from complementary alternative remedies.

finding an increasingly important place in healing today. The psychological effect of a herbal remedy or just-prepared vegetable soup, served by mother in the comfortable environment of home, does much more than starched white bedsheets in an antiseptically clean, impersonal hospital room, where one's pills are dispensed in a routine manner. However, massage should only be done where suggested in this book. Unsupervised massage can be counter-productive or downright dangerous, as in the case of acute inflammation, abnormal skin conditions, varicose veins, etc.

Hot or Cold Compresses

A small Turkish hand towel, or a handkerchief-sized soft absorbent cloth is soaked in a hot or cold infusion/decoction, wrung out gently, so that all the water is not squeezed out, and the cloth is applied to the affected part of the body. In the case of a hot compress, leave it on till the cloth cools to room temperature. The heat of the cloth, with the medicament, affects the part by increasing the circulation to the area, and the debris of destruction, an aftermath of the battle between the body's defence mechanisms and the offending agent—the metabolic by-products of the inflammatory reaction—are lifted away. The exudate of the swelling is sucked out, thereby lessening the pain. There is no stretch now, so the pain fibres are not stimulated. A cold compress, which one applies in the case of a fresh sprain, helps reduce the swelling. A cold compress also brings the temperature down. A compress of either type needs to be changed frequently when it reaches room temperature, say every 4-5 minutes. The ritual of changing compresses loses its efficacy after 25-30 minutes.

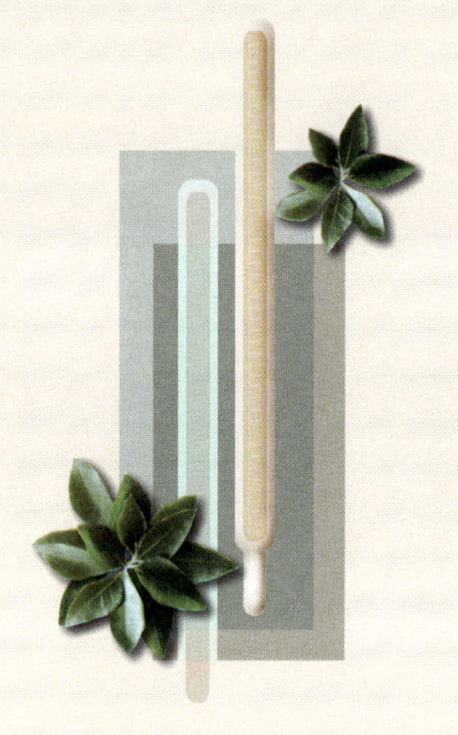

A RISE IN TEMPERATURE
INDICATES THAT SOMETHING IS
WRONG WITH THE BODY.
FEVERS WHICH LAST LESS
THAN A WEEK ARE CAUSED BY
COMMON INFECTIONS. THOSE
WHICH TAKE LONGER TO GET
ALL RIGHT ARE MORE SERIOUS
IN NATURE AND NEED
MEDICAL ATTENTION.

FEVER

The human body has a normal core temperature of 37.0 degrees centigrade or 98.6 degrees fahrenheit. Any variation in this core figure implies that something is amiss. Fever is a protective mechanism of the body—the body's response to tissue injury.

Causes and symptoms

Fever may be caused by infections, mechanical trauma, anaemia, heart attack, stroke, haemorrhage, certain metabolic disorders, arthritic conditions, drug reaction, immune dysfunction or cancer. In fact, anything wrong with the body will trigger this reaction, initiated in a centre located in the hypothalamic region of the brain, called the thermo- regulatory centre. Essentially, fever is a protective mechanism of the body and is actually the beginning of the healing process, carried out by the body's defence mechanisms, rather than a symptom. It helps mobilise the white blood cells of the blood, to actually destroy the invader, and either engulf and ingest it or carry away the debris of destruction, for removal by the kidney. White blood cells or WBCs also form a protective screen by the release of antibodies to counter a subsequent attack.

Usually fever, or pyrexia as it is known in medical terms, is a manifestation of a disordered state in the body, yet there are some normal physiological periods in the body's rhythm when a variation in core body temperature may occur. These are periods following vigorous exercise, the latter half of the menstrual cycle and pregnancy. The normal temperature also varies at different times of the day. It is slightly higher during times of physical activity, and lowest during sleep. Just before the menstrual flow begins, the temperature falls a little, and still further, by as much as a degree, 24-36 hours before ovulation occurs, i.e., between two menstrual flow cycles. After ovulation has occurred, it goes up a little and maintains the same level till the beginning of the next flow. The normal body temperature may also rise a little on an exceptionally hot day.

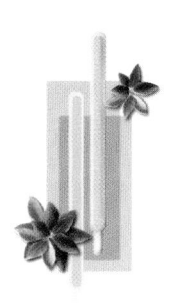

Rise in temperature indicates bodily dysfunction or disorder. Most viral fevers are self-limiting and rarely last more than 3-4 days, e. g., influenza and common cold. Fevers lasting more than a week are caused by less common infections and are likely to be bacterial in nature, e. g., a fever of a duration of more than five days, which rises and falls daily, but never reaches baseline, is likely to be typhoid or paratyphoid. A fever persistently hovering above normal, but never really high enough to need a doctor, may be of tubercular origin, or due to an undiagnosed neoplastic growth. Very high swings in temperature, accompanied by chills and rigors, with the fever abruptly falling, with sweating, may point towards malaria. Febrile states alternating with afebrile or no-fever states, the intervals being 1-2 days, may also be due to lesser-known infections of the Borrelia species.

Most fevers caused by seasonal, mild viral infections can be safely handled at home. However, there are some mild, undiagnosed, low-grade fevers which occur in young women, which do respond to home remedies, but recur again and again. These do not have a disturbing general state accompanying them. Watch out for them, as they may well be the sporadic sub-clinical signs of underlying urinary-tract infection. High fevers cause dehydration—the excessive sweating causes loss of salt, water and vital electrolytes. Fevers higher than 40 degrees centigrade may cause mental confusion, twitching, tremors, delirium and convulsions.

Remedies

■ Bed rest: Rest a fever is an oft-forgotten piece of advice from grandmother. In a fever, the body's defence mechanisms come into play and need a helping hand.

■ Fever should be suppressed only if it goes above 39 degrees centigrade or 101 degrees fahrenheit. If the fever is high, apply cold compresses on the forehead, and sponge the whole body with tepid water. You can add a few drops of eu de cologne, lavender leaves, or a gentle soothing perfume to the water used. This takes away the sour smell of fever. Do not bring down the temperature rapidly, as this confuses the body's temperature regulating centre, causing the body to go into shock. This can be dangerous.

■ Give plenty of fluids orally. Fever, especially high fever, causes dehydration, as mentioned earlier. Go slow on food—a day of fasting helps. In most fevers there is an initial loss of appetite, as the body is using all its energy to combat the cause of the fever. As soon as the temperature comes down, appetite returns. In some not very high but persistent fevers, loss of appetite continues. This, in turn, depletes the body's glucose energy sources. Hence, fruit juices and vegetable soups are ideal nourishing diets to feed a person with fever. The food should be easily digestible—light soft food. *Congee,* a very thin rice gruel seasoned with a flavouring of garlic, with salt to taste, is a favourite in South India—it replenishes lost strength, and brings back appetite in febrile conditions.

■ The leaves of the holy basil plant lead the home herbal list as a febrifuge. The leaves of this plant not only bring down temperature but relieve pain, clear respiratory passages of congestion, and flush out the kidneys. Its anti-inflammatory and analgesic properties are well researched and documented. Holy basil leaves are excellent as a preventive and curative remedy for seasonal fevers.

■ To one-and-a-half teaspoons of dried holy basil-leaf powder, add an equal amount of dried ginger powder; brew with a glassful of water to make a soothing

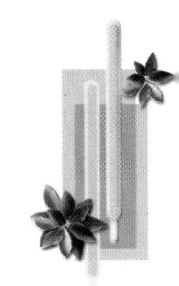

FOR AN ACUTE FEVER OF UNKNOWN ORIGIN, MAKE A DECOCTION WITH 100 GMS OF FRESH HOLY BASIL LEAVES (APPROXIMATELY A HANDFUL) WITH HALF A LITRE OF WATER. THE DECOCTION WILL BE ABOUT THREE-FOURTH OF A CUP. KEEP ASIDE. DIVIDE INTO DOSES—A DECOCTION IS MUCH STRONGER THAN A HERBAL TEA. FOR AN ADULT, GIVE TWO TEASPOONSFUL 3-4 TIMES A DAY; A CHILD OF 6-12 YEARS, A TEASPOONFUL 3-4 TIMES A DAY; A CHILD OF 2-6 YEARS, HALF TO THREE-FOURTH TEASPOONFUL 3-4 TIMES A DAY; A BABY OF 4-12 MONTHS, ONE-FOURTH TO ONE-THIRD TEASPOONFUL THRICE A DAY. TO MAKE IT PALATABLE, ADD MILK, A PINCH OF GREEN CARDAMOM POWDER AND SUGAR TO TASTE. FOR A BABY, THE REMEDY CAN BE GIVEN WITH BREAST MILK—EXPRESS MILK INTO A TABLESPOON, ADD ONE-FOURTH TO ONE-THIRD TEASPOON OF THE DECOCTION, MIX AND FEED DROP-WISE THRICE A DAY. MAKE A FRESH DECOCTION EVERY DAY. THIS IS ALSO EFFECTIVE IN MALARIAL AND DENGUE FEVERS.

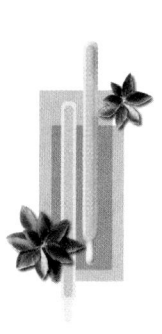

tea. Add sugar and milk to taste. Have three to four times a day. Fresh ginger and holy basil leaves can also be used, but they need to be boiled a little longer to make a decoction. These are especially good for influenza, common cold and all respiratory-tract infections; though they will bring down fever due to any cause. If there is an accompanying cough, add a few ground peppercorns. If the cause is self limiting, 2-3 days' administration will cure the condition. However, chronic conditions will need simultaneous investigation and supervised, specific medical treatment.

■ A standard mixture, very effective by itself, or as a complementary remedy for bronchitis, tuberculosis, cancer of the lungs and gastro-intestinal problems, is made by boiling two cups of dried Indian gooseberry with four cups of water, till just a cup remains. Strain this and keep aside. To this add a level teaspoon each of dried powdered ginger, coriander seeds, cummin seeds, black pepper, long pepper, cloves, cardamoms and cinnamon. Boil this mixture again for a couple of minutes, stirring continuously. Make a syrup, using a cup of sugar for a cup of water, till it is of a one-thread consistency. Add this to the condiment/spice mixture. Boil it again. Now add a cupful of melted ghee, made from cow's milk butter. Stir well till the mixture is well-blended. Cool and store in a clean, dry glass container in a cool, dry place. A level teaspoon of this mixture, taken twice a day, is a keen appetite stimulant, a good digestive, and rich in vitamin-C; plus the active principles released clear the respiratory passages of phlegm and blockages.

■ For suspected malarial fever, a decoction can be made with two tablespoons of the pounded bark of the neem tree, two tablespoons of pounded coriander seeds, and a teaspoon of cardamom. Add to this two glasses of water, bring it to the boil and simmer for half an hour. Adult dose—four teaspoonsful thrice a day. To mask the bitterness of neem, add honey or sugar to taste.

■ Another variation of this basic neem fever potion is two teaspoons each of pounded neem bark, pounded cloves and pounded cinnamon. Mix well, add two glasses of water, and boil for 15 minutes. Strain through a clean muslin cloth and dispense an adult dose of four teaspoonsful thrice a day.

■ A herbal tea is prepared by boiling 8-10 leaves of holy basil with 3-4 fresh,

FENNEL

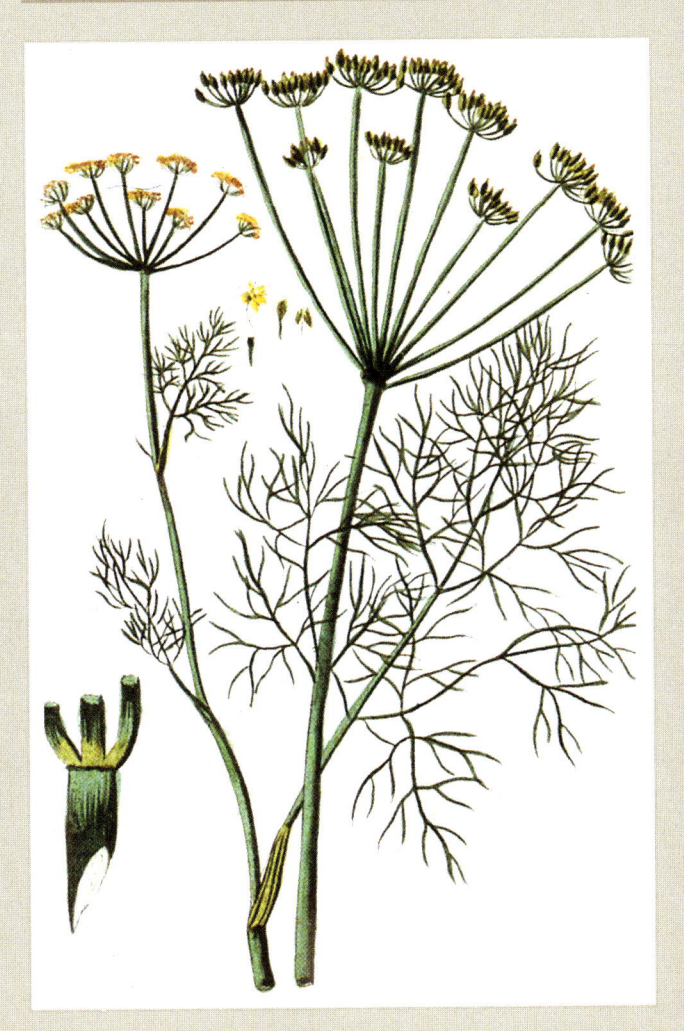

Botanical name:
Foeniculum vulgare

Description and uses: Fennel is a hardy umbeliferous plant with yellow flowers and feathery leaves. Its seeds are dried and used as a food flavouring as well as a remedy for various ailments—the leaves and root are also utilised. Fennel is efficacious for many health problems, and it is used to treat respiratory and gastro-intestinal disorders, hypertension, coughs, hoarseness, persistent indigestion, flatulence, dyspepsia, diarrhoea, colic, biliousness, constipation, dysentery and diabetes.

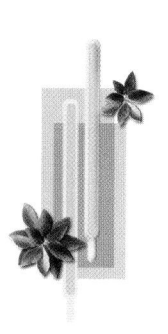

soft, new leaves of the jambul tree in a cup of water. Cooled and sweetened with honey, this is a soothing, refreshing drink, and lowers the temperature in malarial and heat-stroke fevers.

- Fevers caused by gastro-intestinal problems and respiratory infections respond well to a teaspoonful of turmeric powder added to a glass of hot milk with sugar to taste. If there is also constipation, add a teaspoon of hot ghee (clarified butter), stir it well, and while it is still quite hot, drink it in one go. Turmeric has a tendency to settle down in the tumbler, so if you want to sip this drink, keep stirring it. The medicament in the turmeric should get into your system and not remain as dregs at the bottom of the cup!

- Patients with diarrhoea, dysentery, and fever, especially those occurring in summer, should be given *bael* sherbet, alternating it with the holy basil fever potion. This is prepared by mixing the pulp of three ripe *bael* fruits in two glasses of water. Add sugar to taste. Adult dose: four tablespoonsful 3-4 times a day. Give the patient plenty of water to drink, spaced out in between these periods.

- Fenugreek tea: Half a teaspoon of fenugreek seeds, boiled with a cupful of water, cooled, and flavoured with a teaspoon of lemon juice with honey/sugar added to taste, removes the foul sour taste in the mouth and the unpleasant body odour associated with some fevers.

- Mint: Take a handful of crushed fresh mint leaves, 2-3 black peppercorns, 2-3 long peppers, a one-fourth-inch piece of ginger, ground to a fine paste. Boil it in two cups of water. Once it comes to the boil, simmer it for 12-15 minutes. The cooled, filtered mixture, divided into three doses and sipped as a herbal tea, gives relief in fevers associated with gastro-intestinal disorders.

- A decoction made with two tablespoons of fennel boiled with a cup-and-a-half of water, which is reduced to three-fourth of a cup, and a tablespoonful of this taken twice a day, helps in respiratory and gastro-intestinal fevers.

- Suspected typhoid fever can be treated with a decoction made by boiling 10 grams of sisymbrium irio with 10 grams raisins in a litre of water. Boil till it is reduced to one third of the original quantity. This can be given with other medicines.

NEEM

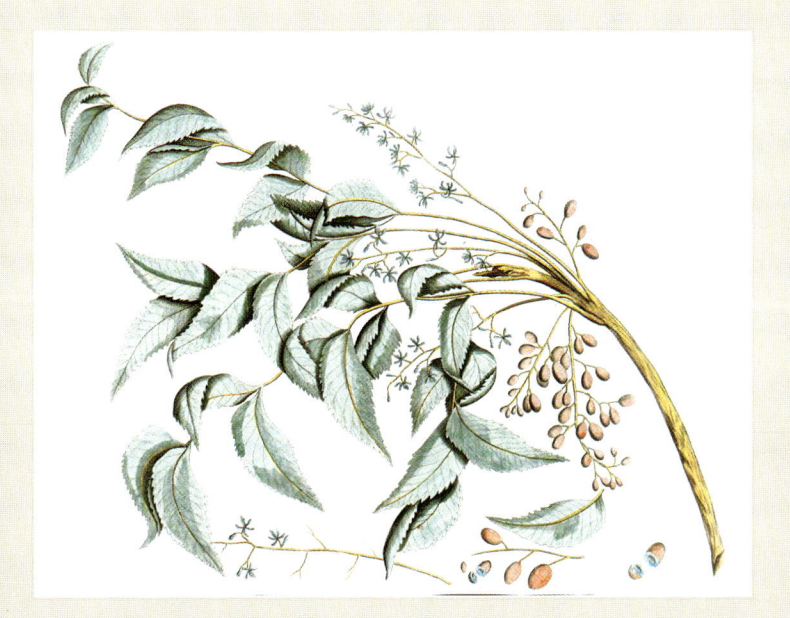

Botanical name: *Azadirachta indica*

Description and uses: The neem tree grows luxuriously in India to a height of 30 to 50 feet, the leaves are bipinnate and the large bunches of lilac flowers are pleasantly perfumed.

Every part of this tree is used and has antiseptic qualities. Special oils prepared from the leaves and seeds are used to treat leprosy and other skin diseases such as eczema, ringworm and scabies. Dandruff is cured by using water with neem leaves as a rinse. The tender twig of the tree is used as a toothbrush to clean the teeth. Neem leaves, fruits and the bark are used to treat fevers, sore throats, earache, mouth ulcers, gingivitis, cholera, intestinal worms, diabetes, measles, chicken pox, heat rash, prickly heat, boils, abscesses, pimples, hair problems and lice.

SAGE

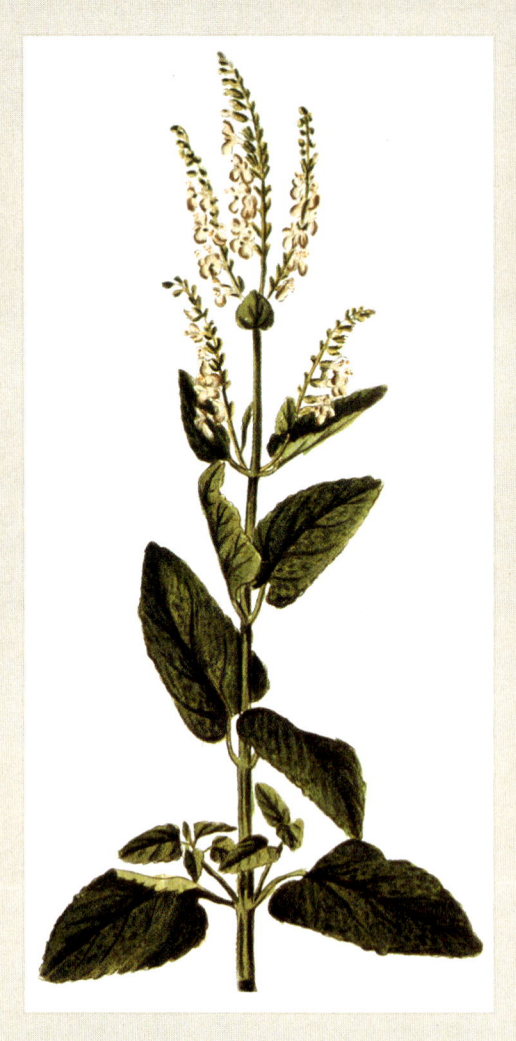

Botanical name: *Salvia officinalis*

Description and uses: It is an aromatic herb with dull greyish-green leaves. Sage generally grows about a foot or more high and has wiry stems. The leaves are set in pairs on the stem, and are one-and-a-half to two inches long, stalked, oblong, rounded at the ends, with a strongly-marked network of veins on both sides and softly hairy and glandular beneath.

Sage has been cultivated for culinary and medicinal puposes for centuries. The name of the genus, *salvia,* is derived from the Latin salvere, to be saved, in reference to the curative properties of the herb. 'Sage helps the nerves by its powerful might, palsy is cured and fever put to flight' is a translation from an old French saying. Sage tea or infusion brings down delirious fever caused by heat and those fevers associated with brain-related and nervous diseases. It is also a stimulant tonic for weakness of digestion. A cup of strong sage infusion relieves nervous headaches and a sore throat, and the fresh leaves, rubbed on the teeth, clean them and strengthen the gums. It is a miraculous cure for a wide variety of illnesses.

■ Malarial fevers respond well to a herbal tea made with chiretta leaves or stems, whether fresh or dried, with honey added to mask the bitter taste. These are usually available in their dry form at the grocery shop. This remedy does not have the side effects of quinine. The stomach tolerates it well, especially if it is mellowed with a dash of honey. However, an overdose causes sickness and a feeling of heaviness in the stomach. These plants grow wild in gardens in the northern and north-eastern regions of India. A teaspoonful of dried leaves or plant powder, made into a decoction, can be taken thrice a day. If it is growing in your garden, use a tablespoon of crushed leaves. Malarial fever also comes down with a lesser-known remedy—the leaves of the coral jasmine or night jasmine. Its flowers are white, with a corolla which is saffron in colour. It has a pleasant fragrance and is usually offered in Hindu temples to the deities. The leaf has antipyretic properties.

■ The best herbal treatment for malaria is a tea made with 12 grams of dried holy basil leaves and 3 grams of black pepper powder, taken thrice a day. Honey, palm candy or sugar are optionals which can be added for taste.

■ For a fever caused by a hot day out in the sun, or during delirium associated with certain fevers of the nervous system, an infusion of fresh sage leaves is very soothing. At the same time, sage tea is highly beneficial in typhoid fever, fever with cold in the head, a sore throat, a peri-tonsillar abscess also known as 'quinsy,' measles, joint pains, and biliousness associated with liver complaints. To make sage tea, put 25 grams sage leaves in a pan, and pour a litre of boiling water over it. Cover and keep aside to cool. When cool, add three tablespoons of fresh lime juice and two tablespoons of honey. Stir and serve cold 3-4 times a day.

■ Tamarind sherbet: Take one tablespoonful of fresh, thick tamarind extract. Add a glassful of boiling water to it. Cool, strain and add sugar to taste. You can have it fairly chilled if you like. It brings down fever speedily in summer.

■ Lemon-grass tea, with honey to taste, is a refreshing remedy for fever.

■ In high fever, the application of cool sandalwood paste on the forehead brings the temperature down, just like a cold compress does.

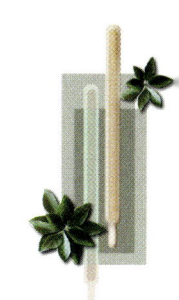

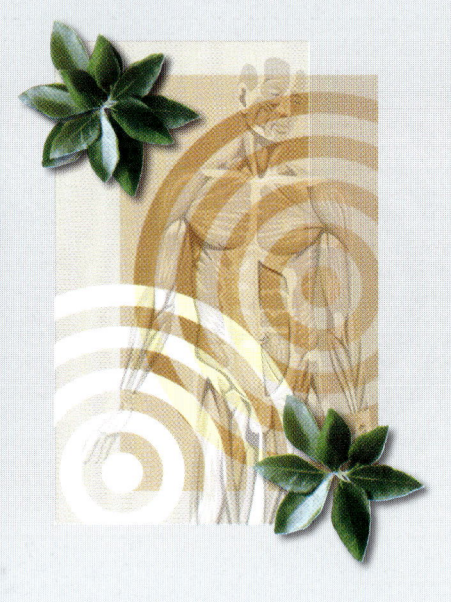

Pain is physically and emotionally distressing for anyone, and is a warning that something is wrong. People differ in their ability to bear pain, but eventually almost everyone seeks help to get to the root of the problem and cure it.

PAIN

What is pain? Pain is an emotionally and physically disturbing, distressing sensation which signals that something is wrong.

Causes and symptoms

Pain is caused by the stimulation of specific nerve endings in the skin and the lining of internal organs. The sensation of pain is the same, whether it is in response to the stimulus of injury, stretching, rise in temperature, loss of blood, or the impending cessation of cellular activity due to damage of any kind in the region. The interpretation of this complexity of reasons is a function of the higher centres in the brain. The sensation of pain is only felt when the nervous impulse transported from an injured or stretched area reaches the brain and is translated into conscious feeling. The degree of pain felt by a person is no indication of the extent of injury, the depth of painful stimuli, the amount the lining covering an organ is stretched, the amount of blood lost in the area, etc. It can be described as soreness, an ache, a mild tenderness, a constriction, a burning, boring or agonising sensation. Depending on one's tolerance to pain, a person seeks relief sooner or later. Examples of pain are dealt with under separate headings—headache, backache, pain in the abdomen. etc., and remedies have been prescribed for the specific site/cause of pain.

Remedies

Most pains respond to rest. Once the cause has been identified, one can try and set the problem right with the resources available.

■ Relaxation: Mental relaxation and coming to terms with the cause of the pain releases certain bio-chemicals in the brain called endorphins. These are pain relievers. The application of a cold compress makes one feel better.

■ Local application of a paste made of henna leaves or flowers is soothing.

■ Holy basil herbal tea has good analgesic properties.

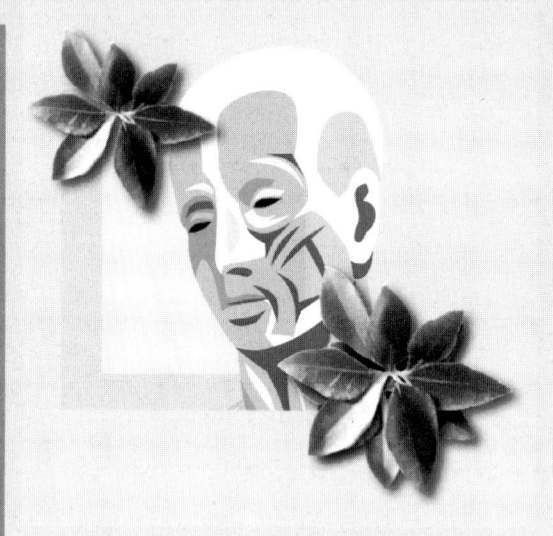

The head houses the brain, which is probably the most vital organ in the body. Therefore, any problem related to the head, whether it is a headache or a head injury, should be immediately attended to and treated.

■ Head-related problems

Head-related problems are very common and most people do not know what to do about them—whether they are headaches or a head injury of any kind. However, they should never be neglected and should be immediately attended to.

HEADACHE

Many people suffer from headaches, and so often, that one wonders whether to treat it with over-the-counter medicines, which may or may not give relief, or just ignore it, hoping it will go away.

Headache is pain in the region of the head. This actually means the brain, which is lodged within the bony skull. The brain, however, has no pain fibres. Hence, if a surgeon used local anaesthesia to make a small incision and proceeded to work on the brain, the patient would feel no pain. However, the membranous covering of the brain, and the walls of the blood vessels supplying it, have a large number of nerve fibres which carry the sensations of touch and temperature. This is felt as pain. So a headache is a warning that something is wrong. The body has an in-built, warning system for timely disaster prevention, and if this works efficiently it has more than a fair chance of controlling the damage. But how many of us recognise an emergency and take suitable action?

Causes and symptoms

A headache could be caused by a late night, having too much to drink, or it may be because of an uncomfortably warm day. The latter results in dehydration without one being aware of it. Pressure of work, emotional stress, mental tension, indigestion, constipation are common but easily missed reasons. But sometimes the cause may be sinister, for example, meningitis, undiagnosed hypertension, or a small stroke in the brain. Missing a meal or skipping meals to lose weight—quite common these days—results in a fall in optimum blood-sugar levels, thereby precipitating a headache. This also happens when a diabetic has his medicine, but inadvertently delays his meal. A headache often heralds the onset of seasonal fevers or infections. Eyestrain, the wrong power in spectacle lenses, incorrect posture, over-strenuous exercise, spondylitis, uneven alignment of the upper and lower jaw, resulting in an uneven bite, or plain unconscious grinding of teeth due to suppressed tensions, all cause headaches. Fluctuating hormones during the puberty years, premenstrual tension or menopausal discomfort cause headaches in women.

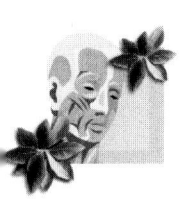

An unilateral headache—when only one side of the head hurts intensely, with nausea, vomiting, visual disturbances, or seeing flashing lights in front of the eyes—is called migraine. Anger, anxiety, excitement or depression, dietary indiscretions or allergy to certain foods often precipitate headaches. Consuming too much caffeine in coffee, tea, cola, etc., can also alter the blood flow to the brain and cause a headache. Strong perfumes can bring about a headache too.

A minor headache can be treated safely with household remedies. But if a headache occurs without any apparent reason, and is associated with a feeling of intense weakness, a sinking sensation, visual complaints, nausea or vomiting, loss of sensation or motor function in any part of the body, never treat yourself at home. Visit the doctor immediately.

Note: *Headache following a head injury, however small and insignificant, with no apparent external signs, must be attended to by a doctor. It may be the first sign of internal haemorrhage inside the skull, or worse.*

Remedies

■ Local applications or a massage helps. A headache caused by being out in the sun will improve by applying a cold compress on the forehead. Adding a few drops of eau de cologne to it will further enhance its efficacy.

For headaches caused by heat and over-exposure to the sun:
■ Lemon peel or orange peel, pounded to a paste with water and applied on the forehead is extremely relaxing and soothing in summer.

■ Holy basil leaves pounded with sandalwood powder, made into a paste with water, and applied on the forehead following sunstroke gives immense relief.

A COLD COMPRESS SOAKED IN AN INFUSION MADE FROM ANY OF THE FOLLOWING—MARIGOLD FLOWERS, ROSE PETALS, LAVENDER, LEMON, ORANGE PEAL, MINT, SAGE, FENNEL OR CLOVES—IS PARTICULARLY SOOTHING.

- A paste of 10-12 cloves and a few small crystals of normal salt with milk can also be applied on the forehead to relieve a headache.

- Very cold weather, or being exposed to a blast of cold wind, can be the cause of a headache, a precursor to a cold. The application of a paste of cinnamon and warm water on the temples and forehead induces a feeling of warmth and aborts a headache. However, it should be done early enough before the cold takes hold.

- Headache associated with cold benefits from inhalation of a rosemary-leaf infusion.

- Take a tablespoon of omum seeds, grind them and make a paste with water. Place in a muslin pouch. Place the pouch in 3/4 litres of boiling water and inhale. This must be done for at least 3-4 minutes.

- A headache caused by a cold coming on is relieved by a herbal tea made from an infusion of holy basil leaves, and if the throat feels sore, alternate it with a warm herbal mixture made with a level teaspoon of fresh ginger juice mixed with a spoonful of honey in hot water, thrice a day. Another effective remedy is a level teaspoon of ground long pepper, with jaggery to sweeten the taste, thrice a day with warm or hot water.

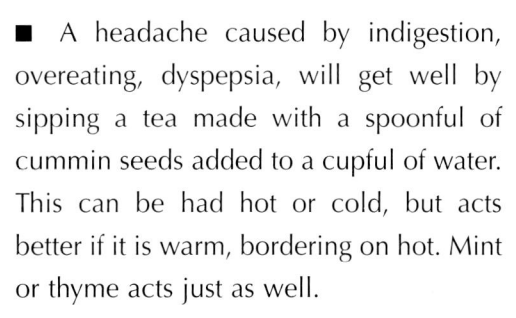

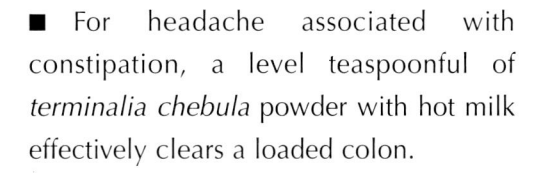

- A headache caused by indigestion, overeating, dyspepsia, will get well by sipping a tea made with a spoonful of cummin seeds added to a cupful of water. This can be had hot or cold, but acts better if it is warm, bordering on hot. Mint or thyme acts just as well.

- For headache associated with constipation, a level teaspoonful of *terminalia chebula* powder with hot milk effectively clears a loaded colon.

- Aloe grows wild in most places with sandy soil in India. Its leaves have many medicinal properties. Dried leaves can be powdered and stored. Take two pinches or one-fourth of a teaspoon of this powder, mixed with an equal amount of turmeric, dissolved in half a cup of water, and drink it. It is especially good for headache complaints associated with menstruation.

- Another lesser known remedy is to extract juice from the leaves of the drumstick tree, and put a drop or two of this into the left nostril for a right-sided headache, and into the right nostril for a left-sided one. Folklore medicine advocates the use of every part of this tree, e.g., in the treatment of ascites, where there

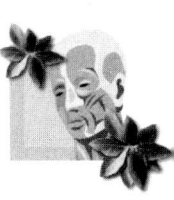

HEADACHES CAUSED BY NERVOUS OR MENTAL STRESS, a result of everyday cares or worries, or just plain overwork, NEED THE INDULGENCE OF A WEEKLY MASSAGE. The rhythmic motion of massage allays joint and muscle stiffness and relaxes the whole body. It brings about a feeling of complete relaxation. Touch is often an unspoken need. It is therapeutic. Some of us need it more than others. Touch make us comfortable living with others. Massage should be done with firm fingers and hands, using pressure which is comfortable, inherently tender for some, and bordering on almost painful for others, without actually being painful.

Massage can be done with or without oil. Sandalwood oil is best for promoting mental balance, a sense of peace and tranquility, and a cool, relaxed mind. However, different people have different temperaments and respond differently to an oil massage. In general, warm mustard or sesame oil have heating properties and are ideal for cold winter days, whereas coconut or olive oil are cooling and can be used in summer. Head massage should be done for at least 10-15 minutes to show any results.

Nervous tension and premenstrual tension headaches are also relieved by a forehead and temple massage with a few drops of crushed marjoram extract, or inhalation from an infusion made from the marjoram plant. It relieves headache because it has a camphoraceous principle in its essential oil—camphor has anaesthetic properties.

Massage the feet with kneading strokes, especially the toes and the area where they join the feet. This exerts pressure on some pressure points and relieves headache. Try it, it works!   A cold compress soaked in an infusion made from any of the following—marigold flowers, rose petals, lavender, lemon, orange peel, mint, sage, fennel or cloves—is particularly soothing.

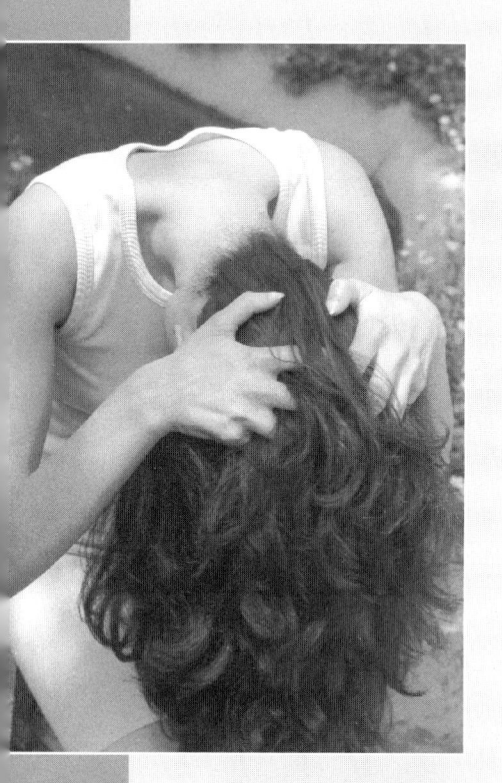

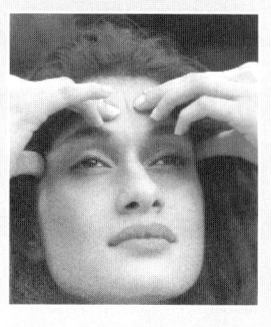

is an accumulation of fluid in the peritoneal cavity, and the abdomen is bloated and distended. This condition is a sequel to serious liver disorder. This remedy relieves unilateral headache probably by regulating the water and electrolyte balance in the inter-and intra-cellular spaces, and in the haemo-dynamics of blood supply to the area.

Prevention

To avoid tension headaches, keep regular hours—eat in time, and never eat in a hurry.
- Get enough sleep.
- Do not bring 'work' tension home.
- Regular exercise (walking, jogging, swimming) will help in relieving stress and tension.
- Avoid drinking too much tea and coffee, and also over-indulging in alcohol and hot, spicy, fried food. For those who have been diagnosed as suffering from migraine, avoid cheese, chocolate, citrus fruits, caffeine and alcoholic drinks, and also port and red wine.
- If possible, learn *pranayam*, the correct way of breathing, from a trained yoga teacher. Or learn *sudarshan kriya*. These will ensure that enough oxygen reaches every cell of your body, which then works to its maximum capacity in a positive manner. Think positive and tension headaches will vanish.

HEAD INJURY

Head injury results in dizziness, headache, inability to focus, and a general feeling of malaise. In some head injuries, there may be a deep cut on the scalp, which bleeds profusely. In others the person becomes unconscious with no apparent external injury.

Remedy

For a small cut on the scalp, apply a clean pressure pad on the wound to stop the bleeding. The scalp skin has hardly any fat under it, so the edges of the wound do not join easily and cause the wound to gape open and bleed. No head injury should be neglected, especially those which appear innocuous, with no apparent external lesion. Patients with a history of a fall, concussion, etc., must be observed for 72 hours at least. Never bandage a head wound tightly or try to remove any embedded foreign material in it. A medical practitioner should deal with it. Any symptom, such as a nose bleed, or bleeding from the ear, is a sinister sign and must be heeded.

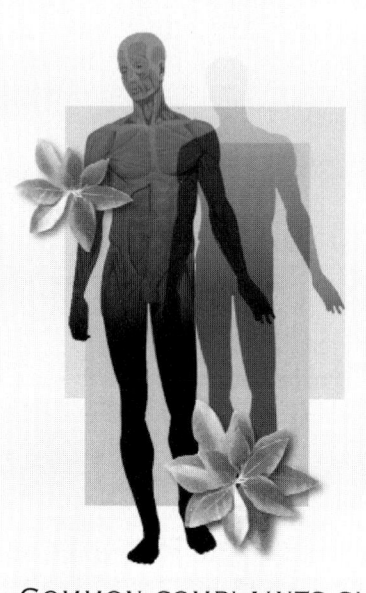

Common complaints such as general weakness, debility, anaemia, nausea and vomiting, dizziness, hypertension, diabetes and depression are often neglected because they are not perceived as serious ailments. However, they need to be treated urgently because they are often caused by underlying and undiagnosed diseases.

GENERAL AILMENTS

There are many health problems which are often neglected and remain untreated. A wide range of ailments come under the category of general ailments. They are the following:

GENERAL WEAKNESS AND DEBILITY

Feeling weak and low on energy is a common complaint experienced by many people today.

Causes and symptoms

The cause may be actual. It could be due to some neuro-muscular disorder, metabolic diseases such as diabetes, deficiency disorders such as anaemia, drug treatment with steroids, or an underlying undiagnosed disease such as cancer, tuberculosis or AIDS. The cause may also be the aftermath of some acute illness such as pneumonia or a viral fever. Weakness and debility following illness causes nutritional deficiency, which leads to depression. It then becomes a vicious circle of depression, loss of appetite, more weakness, and the cycle continues. A feeling of general weakness also results due to over-indulgence in heavy food, smoking, excessive intake of alcohol, narcotic drugs, or even heavy medication. However, it may not be any of these, but a general lack of energy, caused by a sedentary and lazy lifestyle. Sometimes people feel depressed without any reason.

Remedies

■ Avoid spicy, fried foods, and always eat freshly cooked meals. Modern conveniences such as refrigerators, microwave cookers/ovens, cut and polythene-wrapped vegetables, pre-cooked processed foods, to which additives have been added to increase shelf-life, have given rise to people eating food which lack or are deficient in energy-giving vital substances, such as vitamins and trace elements, as well as minerals. Pharmaceuticals race to produce these vital substances in the laboratory in 'better and better forms, with more absorbability'. But there is nothing to beat the form in which they are available in nature.

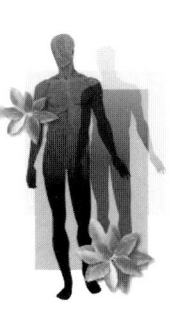

■ Eat plenty of fresh fruits, vegetables and salads. Tonic herbs include parsley, chives, sweet cicely, chervil and asparagus. They are specific for healing and convalescence related to liver/ kidney disorders and arthritis.

■ One-fourth of a teaspoon of cardamom powder in a glass of hot milk, flavoured with a trace of nutmeg or mace, makes a soothing nightcap for people in a debilitated condition or depressed state of mind.

Your diet should include wholegrain cereals and those lentils which contain easy-to-digest protein in them, e. g., alfalfa and mung. Other cooked dried beans are also healthy, but their protein content is much more difficult to digest when one is in a debilitated and weak physical condition. The easiest to sprout are mung, alfalfa, chickpea, green lentils and soya bean. Bean sprouts are extremely nutritious and healthy, because, as the beans soaked in water soften due to the water imbibed, and germination begins to takes place, the nutritious stored nutrients such as the oils, fatty acids and starches begin to change form bio-chemically, turning into enzymes, vitamins, simpler proteins and sugars. As soon as the water is removed, and they are left in a moderately warm and dark place, roots form, and in 2-3 days tender, green shoots sprout. All these sprouts are rich in trace elements and minerals which they imbibe from the atmosphere around them, e.g., the vitamin-C content of a bean sprout is more than 500 times what it contains in its seed state.

Note: A word of caution—high-protein beans, like soya beans, must be washed gently in the first stage of germination, and then cooked in fresh water before they are eaten. The water in which they have been soaked contains certain metabolic waste products of protein change, which makes them difficult to digest. These waste products are toxic in nature, and need to be removed by rinsing the bean sprouts gently but thoroughly once or twice before cooking it. They may cause allergic reactions in people who suffer from lupus, an auto-immune disorder.

ANAEMIA

Anaemia is not always a diagnosis. It is a name, a label, which brings to our notice that there is an underlying disorder which needs to be identified and treated.

Causes and symptoms

Anaemia is a symptom when the patient looks pale because of a fall in the number of circulating red blood cells in the blood. Blood is not just a fluid present in our blood vessels—it is a vital tissue, a life-sustaining system. Blood gets its colour from the presence of a protein pigment called haemoglobin in a certain fraction of its cellular constituents. This pigment combines with oxygen to give blood a bright red colour. The red blood cells flow in the blood stream and supply oxygen to all body tissues, big and small, right down to the tiniest little cell in the body. This oxygen is vital for the life-sustaining metabolic processes in all cells. When we inhale air, our lungs take in oxygen, which is used at the cell/tissue level. One of the waste products of metabolism is carbon dioxide, which the haemoglobin brings back to the lungs. Carbon dioxide is breathed out with every breath we exhale. If for some reason the red cells in the blood become less in number, e.g., due to haemorrhage, a congenital red cell formation defect, dietary deficiencies, infections or bleeding disorders, etc., more blood is needed to transport the same tissue requirement of oxygen. Since there is no more blood available, the same amount of blood has to make more trips for the same work. So, in such a case the heart beats more often, and the heart rate increases. This increase in the heart rate needs more effort. Normally, one is not aware of one's heartbeat. But the extra effort is consciously felt as palpitations. When the requirement becomes even more, as in severe anaemia, the heart muscle also gets less supply of blood, i.e., less oxygen for its optimal functioning, and there is delay in removing carbon dioxide as well as other waste products bacause of this extra muscular action. So there is pain in the chest, which is called angina.

Anaemia causes marked pallor in a person, breathlessness, increase in heart rate, palpitations, fatigue, restlessness, dizziness, headache, irritability and drowsiness—all the systems are working below par. Women are more prone to anaemia, as they menstruate, and a certain amount of blood is lost every month. They are also prone to anaemia during pregnancy, when the foetus draws nourishment from the mother. This is, however, normally compensated by a healthy diet. In the case of women who suffer from excessive bleeding due to menstrual abnormalities, or have repeated pregnancies without adequate spacing, anaemia sets in early, and its presenting symptoms mimic those associated with heart disease. In such situations, actual heart disease may not be diagnosed, as the attending physician may interpret the symptoms as related to a female disorder.

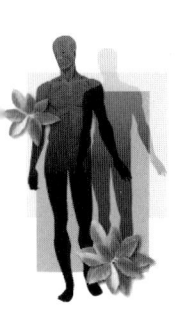

Malnourished children also fall victim to anaemia. Certain drugs prescribed for systemic disease, e.g., anti-malarial drugs, aspirins, sulfonamides, antibiotics such as chloramphenicol, may all cause anaemia. Some people have an enzyme deficiency called G6PD deficiency. This affects certain metabolic processes related to red blood cell formation.

Remedies

- The cause of anaemia needs to be identified and treated. Certain naturally occurring foods help more than others do. For the healthy formation of red blood cells, the body needs protein, iron and trace elements. Wholegrain wheat, rice and other cereals in a vegetarian diet take care of protein needs. It is iron and trace elements which are neglected.

- Almonds are a rich source of iron and trace elements. Soak 8-10 almonds overnight. Next morning peel the almonds, grind them coarsely, mix with a glass of hot milk, add honey or jaggery to taste, and have it as a nutritious morning drink instead of tea. Tea interferes with the absorption of iron, and jaggery is a rich source of iron with some vitamin-B complex too. If you do not like the taste of jaggery in milk, replace it with honey.

- Pistachio is another nut which is extremely rich in iron. In fact, Punjabis and Gujaratis are very fond of milk flavoured with ground masala which contains a mixture of 2-3 almonds, 2-3 pistachos, 2-3 strands of saffron, a pinch each of green cardamom, nutmeg and cinnamon powders. This is a very nourishing nightcap, which ensures a soothing and restful sleep.

- Another healthy drink to be taken during the day, especially in summer, is half a cup of fresh pomegranate juice with a pinch of ground cinnamon powder and a teaspoon of honey once a day. A teaspoon of ground pomegranate seeds can also be had with a cup of milk. It is nourishing and energising.

■ India is a vast country with diverse eating habits. Yet, practically everyone uses fresh coriander leaves daily, either for garnishing, or grinding them with green chillies and various spices, lime or tamarind, coconut, etc., to make chutneys. Ground coriander-seed powder, a condiment used in daily cooking, not only provides fibre in the diet, but also iron and trace elements. Make tea with two teaspoons of coriander powder, boiled in a cupful of water for 2-3 minutes. Strain, cool and add honey and/or milk to taste. Drink twice a day. This tea can be made by replacing coriander with a teaspoon of fenugreek seeds. Fenugreek seeds have a very strong flavour and a slightly bitter taste, hence the quantity used is less.

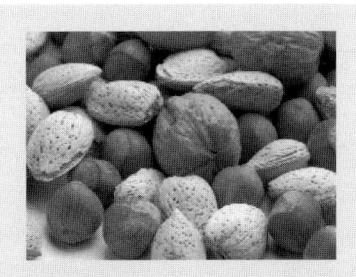

Foods/condiments/spices rich in iron and trace elements, essential as the main or complementary treatment for anaemia are almonds, cashew nuts, dry coconut, sesame seeds, pistachios, asafoetida, cummin seeds, dried mango powder, poppy seeds, tamarind pulp and turmeric; and fruits such as apples, papayas and pomegranates.

NAUSEA/VOMITING

Nausea and vomiting are symptoms of internal disorder, the causes of which are many. Nausea is that queasy feeling in the pit of your stomach which makes you want to throw up, e.g., at the sight of blood, at take off or landing in an aircraft. And, actually throwing up the delicious meal you just had is vomiting.

Causes and symptoms

The ailment may be caused by a throat infection, tonsillitis, if the mucosal lining of the enlarged tonsils is inflamed, and anything swallowed, even saliva, may irritate the nerve endings, causing nausea or actual vomiting. Hepatitis is another cause, where, depending on the extent and seriousness of the cause, there may be slight nausea or actual persistent vomiting. Certain drugs/ prescribed medications, chemotherapy, systemic infections, poisoning, travel sickness, emotional upsets or stress, are some of the other causes. Simple causes, which are not life-threatening, such as morning sickness during early pregnancy, or the sight of blood, or seeing a reptile, may be simple and easy to treat. But persistent, unprovoked vomiting needs specific investigation. Whatever the cause, it needs to be discovered and treated. Meanwhile, there is the urgent need to settle that queasy feeling and to prevent dehydration by replacing vital fluids and essential electrolytes lost.

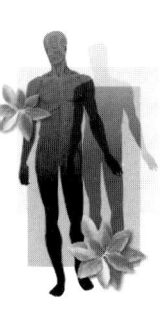

Remedies

■ Simmer a small piece of crushed ginger and a few basil leaves in a cupful of water. Strain the mixture, add honey, and sip hot or cold, as you prefer. Drink a total of half to three-fourth of a cup at a time, but do not drink it all in one go. Gulping the mixture will cause vomiting again.

■ Mint tea, with two ground cloves and a trace of nutmeg is also soothing and leaves a pleasant taste in the mouth.

■ An infusion of curry leaves or sipping fresh, not too sour buttermilk, seasoned with curry leaves, to which a little salt and sugar is added, is a settling, soothing, refreshing and rehydrating drink.

■ Tea made with a handful of fresh, tender, crushed *bael* leaves, sipped half a cup at a time, 2-3 times a day, also settles the stomach. Honey/sugar/jaggery/palm candy can be added for taste. This drink is very nourishing too.

■ The bark of the curry-leaf tree has many medicinal properties. Dried bark can be powdered and stored. Half a teaspoon of the bark powder, taken with cold water, helps greatly in nausea or vomiting due to bilious disorders, hepatitis, etc.

■ Another preparation to make and store is grated fresh ginger, rolled in salt and sun-dried—the extra salt can be dusted off when dry. Just keeping a little of this concoction in the mouth, and gently chewing it, lessens the feeling of nausea.

■ Soak cummin seeds overnight in water with a little lime juice and salt. Next morning, put it out in the sun to dry. Repeat this drying exercise daily till the seeds are completely dry. Store in a clean, dry, airtight container. This too relieves nausea and vomiting when half a teaspoonful is kept in the mouth. You can chew this—it will not harm you. In fact, this remedy and the one before this stimulates the production of saliva, which should be swallowed. Sipping water with either of these in the mouth leaves a clean, sweet taste in the mouth.

- Combat dehydration by drinking enough water. Do not gulp water, as it will set off reverse peristalsis. Just sip whatever fluids you like the taste of and feel you can hold in your stomach. This water is in addition to any of the remedies mentioned above. If you vomit more than once, then for every glass of water you drink add a level teaspoon of sugar or jaggery and a pinch of salt. If there is diarrhoea along with the vomiting, the fluid intake should be at least 6-8 glasses a day.

Note: *If the vomiting is profuse, persistent, or has blood in it, go to a hospital immediately. Lightheadedness, increase in thirst, and decrease in urinary output implies that dehydration has set in, and there is no time to lose. Dehydration can only be combated with fluid replacement, either orally or intravenously.*

DIZZINESS AND FAINTING

A sudden transient impairment of consciousness, not amounting to actual loss of consciousness, where there is an inability to maintain postural tone, is dizziness or feeling faint.

Cause and symptoms

This is caused by impaired blood supply to the brain, resulting in an inability to maintain one's posture. Falling down involuntarily, or consciously lying down when one feels faint ensures that cerebral blood flow is resumed. Impaired blood supply may be caused by simple causes such as standing in the sun too long, a sudden emotional shock, the sight of blood or even a hypodermic needle, trauma, minor surgery, missing meals, dieting or starvation. Sometimes getting up suddenly from a recumbent state may precipitate a fainting episode. This is called postural or orthostatic hypotension. Other causes include prescription drugs such as anti-hypertensives, nitrates, vasodilators or diuretics. Usually when a fainting episode is about to take place, there is a slight feeling of disorientation and one becomes aware that something is not quite right—one tries to grasp and hold on to something or someone, to try and save oneself from falling. When this happens, with absolutely no warning, or a feeling of disorientation, the episode is referred to as a syncope or syncopial attack. Repeated attacks of dizziness or fainting need proper investigation and subsequent treatment. Anaemia, cardiac and circulatory disorders are the common culprits, but epilepsy, Parkinsonism and cerebro-vascular problems are other worrying reasons.

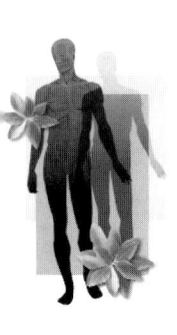

Remedies

■ Do not crowd around the patient. Loosen all tight-fitting clothing.

■ Herbal teas made with a pinch of finely ground cinnamon, or a few crushed, fresh leaves of mint, sage or rosemary, or just plain lemon juice and honey, are good restoratives.

HYPERTENSION

A rise in blood pressure above the normal is referred to as high blood pressure or hypertension. But what is blood pressure?

Blood is a fluid medium—a vital tissue system with certain cellular elements which have specific functions. A certain faction carries oxygen and other essential nutrients to body cells, near and far. Another faction looks after the defence and immunity against infections. While yet another ensures that haemorrhage is controlled in time and a person does not bleed to death. To carry this blood to its destination, there are blood vessels; and the pressure exerted by the flow of blood against the vessel wall during its transit is called blood pressure. This pressure is caused by the force of contraction, which the heart muscle exerts to pump the blood out of the heart. The elasticity of the vessel wall sustains the onslaught of the pressure. Blood pressure is determined by the force of the contraction of the heart muscle, the resistance or elasticity of the vessel wall, the quantity of blood being pumped from the heart into the vessels, and lastly the viscosity of the blood. The latter depends upon the cellular or fluid constituents which make up the blood volume.

GINGER

Botanical name:
Zingiber officinale

Description and uses: Ginger is a perennial root which creeps and spreads underground in tuberous joints. It sends up from its roots a green reed with narrow, lanceolate leaves. The root is used after the plant dies. Ginger has a penetrating and aromatic odour, and its taste is spicy and biting. It is used to treat nausea and vomiting, colds, chest problems, toothache, hyperacidity and heartburn, indigestion, dyspepsia, biliousness, stomachache, diarrhoea, flatulence, constipation, biliousness and loss of appetite in jaundice, piles, kidney problems, arthritis, sprains and strains, allergic rashes, period pains and scanty periods.

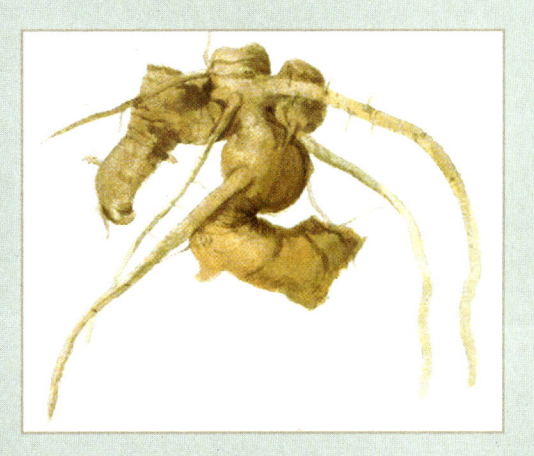

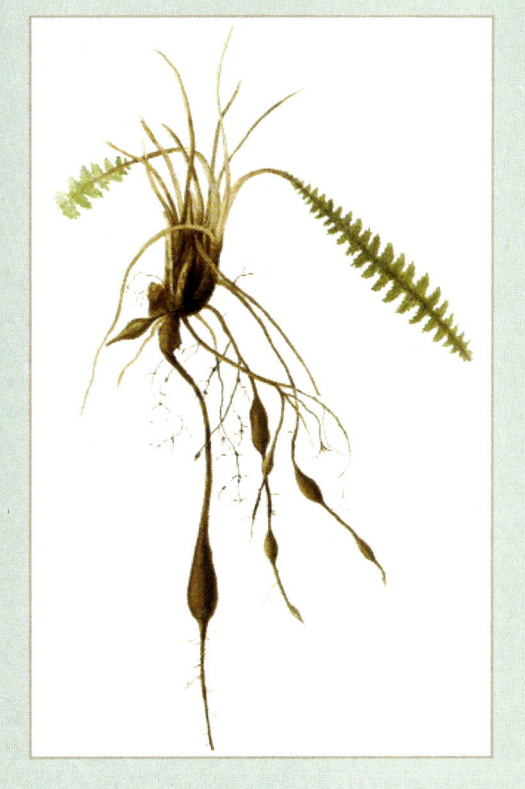

CINNAMON

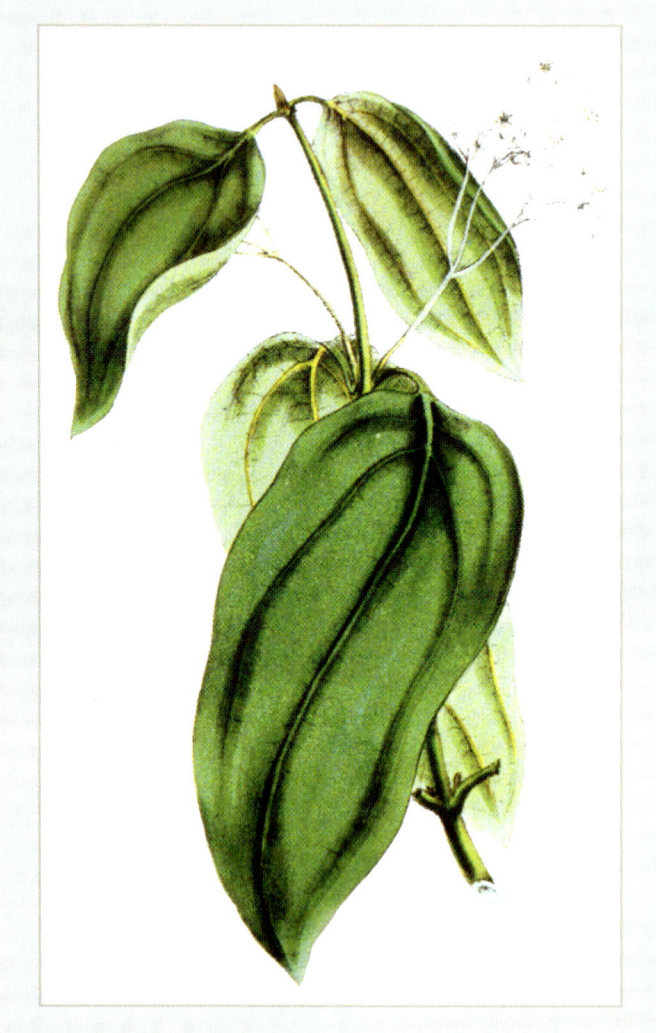

Botanical name: *Cinnamomum zeylanicum*

Description and uses: The cinnamon tree grows to a height of 20 to 30 feet. It has a thick, scabrous bark, strong branches, and the leaves are petiolate. Commercial cinnamon is the dried bark of the tree. It has a fragrant perfume, an aromatic and sweet taste, and is brown in colour.

Cinnamon is carminative, antiseptic, astringent and a stimulant. It is prescribed as an infusion, a paste, and in powder form, often combined with other herbal remedies. It is useful for headaches caused by extreme cold weather and winds; throat problems, including hoarseness; diarrhoea, acne, and any swelling caused by inflammation.

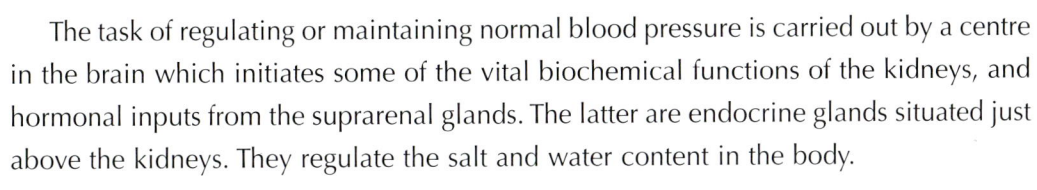

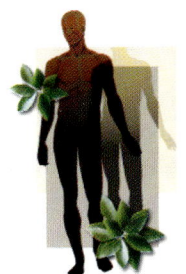

The task of regulating or maintaining normal blood pressure is carried out by a centre in the brain which initiates some of the vital biochemical functions of the kidneys, and hormonal inputs from the suprarenal glands. The latter are endocrine glands situated just above the kidneys. They regulate the salt and water content in the body.

Causes and symptoms

A faulty diet, smoking, emotional upheavals, anxiety and stress are factors which often have a direct bearing on blood pressure. The elasticity of the blood-vessel walls diminishes with age, and certain deposits accumulate on the inner lining. These are worn-out cellular elements and certain cholesterol factions. For some not fully understood reason, some people are genetically predisposed to this condition. They have a familial tendency to certain lipid (fat) metabolic disorders.

High blood pressure in the initial stages usually goes undetected. It is often an accidental finding during a medical check-up for other reasons. However, headaches, fatigue, nosebleeds, shortness of breath, swelling of the feet, palpitations, nervousness are symptoms that warrant the necessity of an early blood-pressure check-up. Depending on one's genetic disposition to high blood pressure, or dietary indiscretions, and the actual blood pressure, certain dietary supplements or restrictions can help keep it in check.

Remedies

■ Boil a cup of water with a teaspoon of dried *bael*-leaf powder. Cool and filter it and drink it thrice a day. *Bael* leaves can be dried, ground in a mixie to a fine powder, and stored in a dry jar. The active ingredient in this powder has natural diuretic properties that helps to regulate blood volume, and hence blood pressure.

■ To prepare another remedy, make a paste using a teaspoon of finely ground cummin seed powder, a pinch of sandalwood powder, two-tablespoons of fresh coconut water, and two tablespoons fresh milk. Mix these together, and add sugar to taste. If you wish to add more coconut water to the mixture you can do so. This should be taken in the morning for a week to 10 days. It has anti-stress, adapto-genic properties, besides being a diuretic.

■ Grind one measure each of fennel, cummin seeds and a small lump of crystallized sugar together, and have a teaspoon of this mixture in the morning and evening after meals. It has ample fibre, which helps to remove the bad cholesterol, and it is also an antiflatulent and diuretic. This remedy is especially beneficial in hypertension associated with pregnancy.

■ A tablespoon of freshly expressed Indian gooseberry juice, sweetened with honey, and taken once in the morning, and half a teaspoon of the dried powder taken with hot water at bedtime, decreases the level of low-density cholesterol, which is instrumental in causing atherosclerotic changes and cholesterol deposits in the inner walls of blood vessels.

■ A glass of fresh orange juice or grape juice, or raw vegetable juice made with carrots and spinach, or a mixture of the two, is extremely beneficial. These juices are rich in beta-carotene, vitamin-C and potassium, which are all beneficial in bringing down blood pressure.

Note: *A word of caution! Those who have hypertension associated with kidney disorders should avoid all these as their high potassium levels are lethal for already disturbed kidney functions.*

■ However, half a teaspoon of the kernel of watermelon seeds, mixed with half a teaspoon of poppy seeds, ground together and taken in the morning and evening for a month, brings down high blood pressure levels. They have no sodium or potassium in them.

■ A decoction of a tablespoon of coriander seeds, with a glass of water, reduced to half, strained and taken twice daily, is a good diuretic as well as a

A LOW-FAT DIET, ESPECIALLY A REDUCTION IN ANIMAL FATS, SUGAR, SALT, REFINED FLOUR, WHITE BREAD, PROCESSED FOODS, ALL HELP IN LOWERING HIGH BLOOD PRESSURE. INCREASING FIBRE IN THE DIET, EATING WHOLEGRAIN CEREALS, AND INCLUDING POTATOES, AVOCADOS, TOMATOES AND LIMA BEANS IN THE DIET PROVIDES A RICH SUPPLY OF POTASSIUM TO THE BODY. THE INTAKE OF LOW-FAT MILK AND YOGHURT, COTTAGE CHEESE, SESAME SEEDS, SPINACH, BROCCOLI AND CHICKPEAS ENSURES AN ADEQUATE AMOUNT OF CALCIUM TO BALANCE THE ELECTROLYTES AT THE CELLULAR BIOCHEMICAL EQUATION LEVEL.

cholesterol-lowering remedy (coriander seeds are very low in potassium).

■ Wash, dry and powder the roots of the holy basil plant. Filter it through a muslin cloth and store it in a dry jar. A pinch of this powder with half a teaspoon of honey, twice a day, helps in keeping high blood pressure in check. Holy basil has anti-stress properties, it 'purifies' the blood by balancing the blood lipid profile, and also acts as a diuretic.

Note: *Continuous or excessive intake of holy basil brings down the sperm count. It also has abortifacient properties.*

■ Another variation of the remedy given above is a mixture of half a teaspoon each of fennel, cummin seeds and granulated sugar. Grind them together. Have twice a day with half a cup of water. This mixture has sedative as well as diuretic properties, and a lot of fibre too, which keeps the lipids in check. It is specially recommended for hypertension associated with pregnancy, and is routinely used by midwives in Indian villages.

■ A herbal drink, which is not cooked, is made with a teaspoon of finely ground cummin seed powder, two tablespoons of

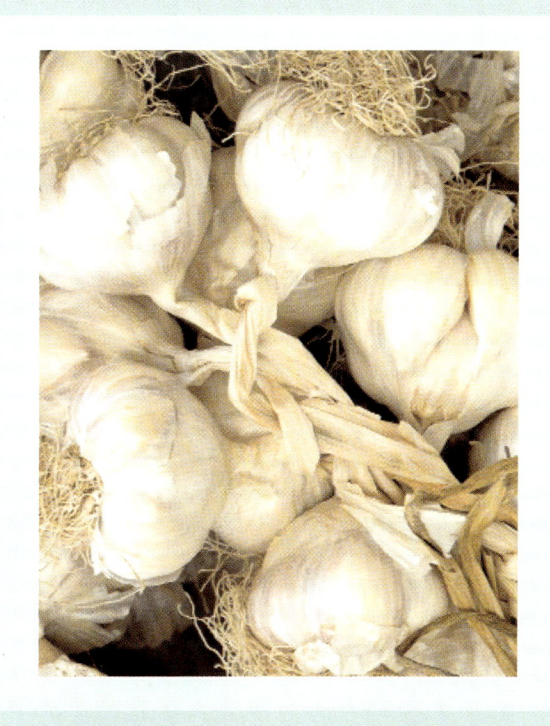

Garlic is another remedy which has no sodium or potassium, but contains certain cholesterol-lowering properties. Two or three cloves or half a teaspoon of garlic powder, taken every day in the morning, is an effective remedy. However, those with weak stomachs or people who are prone to acidity, heartburn or peptic ulcer should avoid this much-publicised-good-for-everything remedy.

milk, two tablespoons of coconut water, and half a teaspoon of sandalwood paste, mixed together. Add water to make half a cup of the drink. Drink it twice a day for a week to 10 days. This has stress-relieving, sedative properties.

■ A tablespoon of freshly expressed Indian gooseberry juice, sweetened with honey and taken in the morning with hot water cools the system. The active ingredients of this mixture are rich in vitamin-C, and also lower the bad cholesterol in the blood, i.e., low-density cholesterol, which is instrumental in causing atherosclerotic changes in the inner walls of the blood vessels.

■ A glass of fresh orange juice or grapefruit juice, or half a cup of raw vegetable juice made with carrots or spinach, or a mixture of the two, is extremely beneficial. These are rich in beta-carotene, vitamin-C and potassium, and are all beneficial in maintaining optimum blood pressure levels.

■ Fresh lime juice with warm water and honey in the morning is another remedy.

Note: All these are good as complementary remedies for hypertension, but are not advised when there is associated kidney disorder. In kidney disorder, there is the need to lower the potassium in the diet, and for hypertension a restricted sodium intake is advised.

The following remedies have a very low sodium and potassium content and a cholesterol-lowering effect:

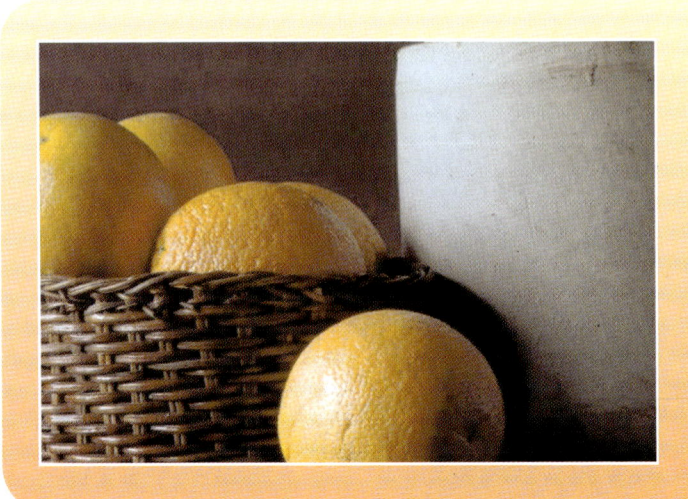

Fresh orange juice therapy, excluding all other food from one's diet for two days, and only drinking fresh (sweet) orange juice will help bring down persistently high levels of blood pressure.

- Half a teaspoon of dry garlic powder, or two cloves of garlic taken daily in the morning lower blood pressure levels. The garlic cloves should be soaked in fresh milk (just enough to cover them) for one hour. They can be chewed or just swallowed, which is much easier to do. However, those with weak stomachs or those prone to acidity, heartburn or peptic ulcers should avoid this much-publicised remedy.

- A decoction of a tablespoon of coriander seeds with a cup of water, reduced to half, strained and taken twice daily, is a good diuretic as well as a cholesterol-lowering remedy.

- Mix a teaspoon of powdered cummin seeds with a teaspoon of fresh ginger juice and a teaspoon of honey. Have this mixture once a day to reduce hypertension.

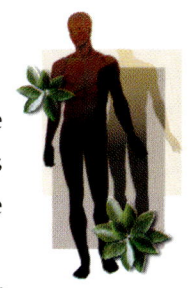

- To a cup of curd, add a medium-sized sliced raw onion, a pinch of turmeric powder, and a clove of lightly roasted, finely chopped fresh garlic. It is good for lowering high blood pressure, and specially beneficial for those who have hyperlipidemia. Onion and garlic both lower lipid levels in blood. In this preparation, only the curd has a little sodium and potassium, whereas onion and garlic have none. Chewing parsley leaves after eating garlic clears the garlic odour from the breath.

- Having a teaspoon of fresh, yellow drumstick-leaf juice after meals is a lesser known remedy for lowering blood pressure. A palatable way of having it is as a chutney. Grind to a fine paste a handful of fresh, well-washed drumstick leaves, a medium-sized onion, a 1/2-inch piece of ginger, and a 1-inch-piece of tamarind (without seeds), with salt and green chillies to taste. This is rich in anti-oxidant beta-carotene, which neutralises free radicals.

> Cummin seeds have a high sodium and potassium content, yet have blood pressure-lowering properties. In traditional or indigenous systems of medicine, it is not the isolated active principle which matters, but the crude extracts which have mutually beneficial applications, as yet not properly understood by western researchers.

GRAPE

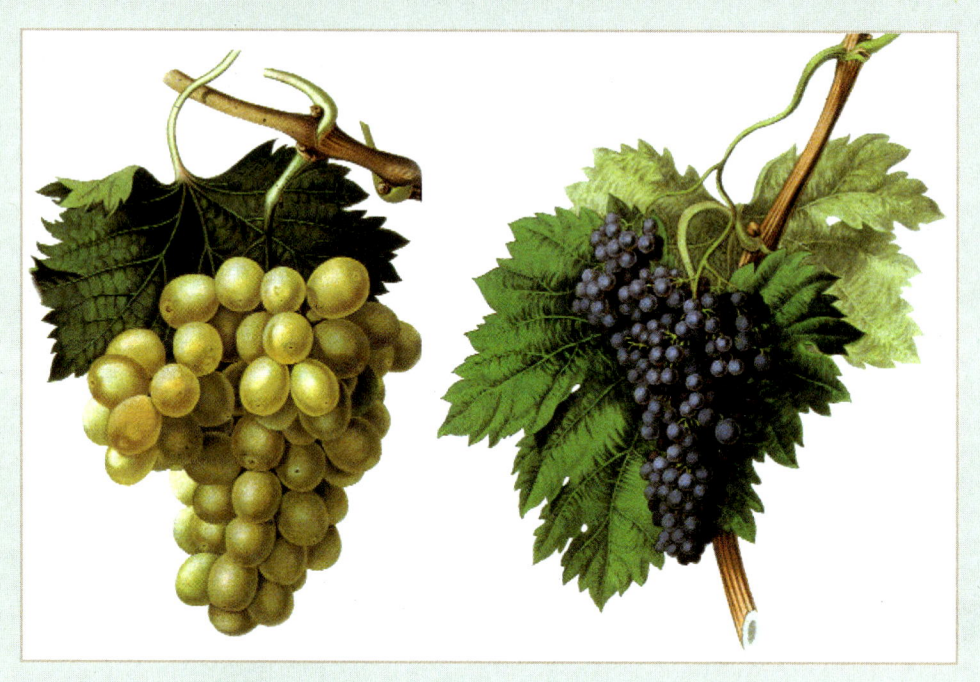

Botanical name: *Vitis vinifera*

Description and uses: Grapes are berries (usually green, purple or black) and grow in clusters on a vine. The name vine is derived from viere (to twist), and refers to the twining habits of the plant.

Grape sugar differs from other sugars chemically. It enters the circulation without any action of the saliva, rapidly increases strength and repairs waste in fevers. The seeds and leaves are astringent. Grapes induce the kidneys to produce a free flow of urine, and have restorative powers in cases of anaemia. They benefit people who are in a state of extreme exhaustion and those suffering from neuralgia, sleeplessness, hypertension, cataract, breathing problems, constipation and coughs.

DIABETES

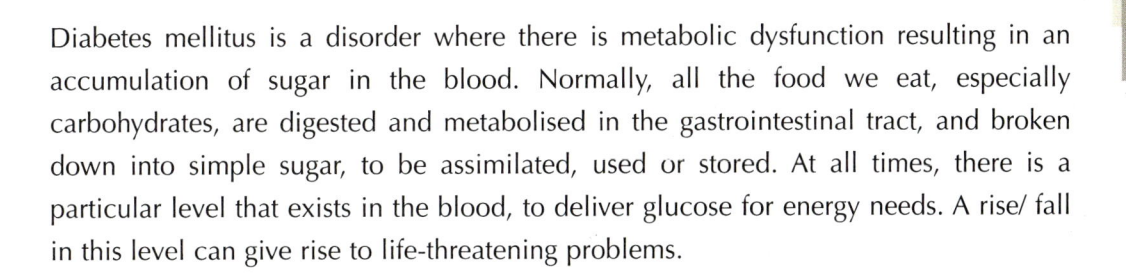

Diabetes mellitus is a disorder where there is metabolic dysfunction resulting in an accumulation of sugar in the blood. Normally, all the food we eat, especially carbohydrates, are digested and metabolised in the gastrointestinal tract, and broken down into simple sugar, to be assimilated, used or stored. At all times, there is a particular level that exists in the blood, to deliver glucose for energy needs. A rise/ fall in this level can give rise to life-threatening problems.

Causes and symptoms

Diabetes mellitus is a condition where the available sugar in the blood is far above normal levels. This can be due to several causes:

- Inadequate insulin, a hormone which is produced by a gland called the pancreas which metabolises sugar and maintains an optimum glucose level in the blood for energy needs.

- It can also be due to the failure of the body to utilise adequately the insulin produced.

- The interplay of the other hormones that indirectly influence the metabolism and utilisation of sugar, e.g., the thyroid, adrenals and pituitary glands.

- The over-production of another hormone from the pancreas which has an effect opposite to that of insulin.

- Viral or bacterial infection or some environmental toxins which damage the pancreas.

Diabetes or its progress finally leads to structural and functional changes in body tissues that are not conducive to meaningful healthy living. Diet plays a very important part in controlling and containing the disastrous effect of this multifaceted metabolic disorder. Professional dietary management needs to be undertaken and followed.

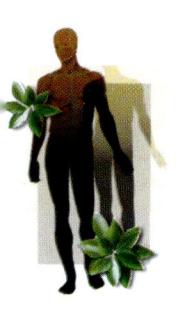

- A genetic predisposition to diabetes.

- The latest finding is that mental or physical stress also causes diabetes or acts as a catalyst in the case of a pre-existing dormant predilection to diabetes.

The main symptoms of diabetes are excessive thirst and appetite, and increased frequency of urination. Other symptoms include wounds not healing, boils, itching in the vulva area, diminishing eyesight, general weakness, etc.

Remedies

The remedies stated below in some cases could control latent diabetes, and in others complement orthodox drug treatment so as to lower the total drug intake. Anyone who is on herbal treatment needs to get his blood sugar checked periodically so that the drug regimen and herb regimen is balanced and the blood sugar does not fall and precipitate another crisis called hypoglycemia—low blood sugar

- The jambul tree's produce heads the anti-diabetic herbal drug list. Numerous scientific studies have been carried out to confirm this.

- The seeds of the jambul have a distinct anti-diabetic action. Dry its seeds, grind, powder and store them. One-fourth of a teaspoon of this powder, taken every morning with a teaspoon of honey, helps to check the excessive conversion of starches into sugar and also helps the inherent insulin in the body utilise sugar better. The jambul pulp per se does not exhibit any significant anti-diabetic action. However, the seeds can bring the blood sugar down by 20 per cent.

- Jambul-seed powder can also be taken with milk. A teaspoonful with half a cup of milk, taken morning and evening, is beneficial.

- Take equal amounts of jambul-seed powder and some home-ground turmeric powder. (The ones sold in the market are processed and lose some of its properties. The rhizome should be dried and powdered). Half a teaspoonful of this mixture should be had with buttermilk or honey twice a day.

- The bark of the jambul tree also has anti-diabetic properties but not as much as the seed. The inner bark of the tree can be dried, burnt to an ash and stored. One level teaspoon of this ash, taken every morning on an empty stomach, and a similar amount an hour after the afternoon and evening meals, helps sugar to metabolise and maintains optimum blood sugar levels conducive to health. Meals should not be missed and should be balanced

- Fenugreek seeds: Fenugreek seeds are a condiment used to season various culinary preparations in meals throughout India. A heaped teaspoonful of seeds soaked overnight in half a cup of water softens them and they become less bitter. Next morning drink this water and eat the seeds with a chapatti or whatever is being eaten for breakfast. This brings down blood glucose levels and reduces cholesterol, especially triglycerides. The seeds can also be eaten without being soaked, but they cause acidity in some people. Soaking the seeds does not change their effect. Ayurveda prescribes remedies depending on the body constitution of a person. The same medicine may have a different effect on different people, hence the correct vehicle is needed. Do not miss meals when taking these medicines, but have them in the correct measure and in time.

- Indian gooseberry: Indian gooseberry plays a vital role in containing diabetes. Take dried Indian gooseberry powder, turmeric and fenugreek-seed powders in equal quantities. Mix and store it. A teaspoon of this mixture taken thrice a day with water is beneficial for early diabetes—keeps it in check.

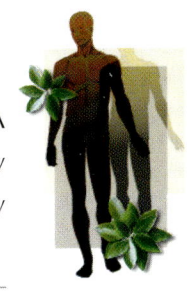

- Take a tablespoon of fresh Indian gooseberry juice, a teaspoon of fresh lime juice, a teaspoon of honey, and add these to a cupful of water. Have every morning on an empty stomach.

- Dried Indian gooseberry powder: Soak a tablespoonful in a cup of water. Next morning filter it. Add half a cup of water, a pinch of ground black pepper and a tablespoon of fresh lime juice to it. Have early in the morning on an empty stomach.

- Bitter gourd is a very popular vegetable in Indian cuisine. Methods for its preparation are varied, but by and large, all the ingredients used help the body utilise sugar well. However, for those with diabetes, having the juice of two large or 3-4 small bitter gourds i.e., about one-third of a cupful daily in the morning, is beneficial. The juice should be extracted from the whole vegetable, including the skin, seeds, inner pulp, etc. Tender green bitter gourds should be cut into small pieces and completely dried in the shade. When dry, powder them fine and store them. A teaspoonful should be had in the morning and evening for at least 3-4 months. It is advised that a constitution identification be done by an expert ayurvedic physician first, as an excess could cause either vomiting or diarrhoea. Besides, some skin aliments already present, not related to the diabetic condition, could get worse. It is a wrongly believed that drinking bitter gourd juice cures all skin aliments.

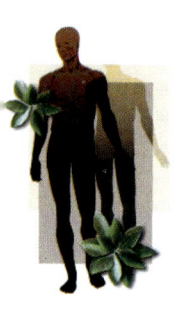

- Two teaspoons of fresh bitter gourd-leaf juice, taken with a large pinch of ground asafoetida every morning, is a lesser-known remedy for diabetes.

- Alternatively, a tablespoon of fresh Indian gooseberry juice, mixed with a tablespoon of fresh bitter gourd juice, taken early in the morning, is also effective.

- Soak a tablespoon of whole black gram dal at night. Next morning drain the water and tie the dal in a damp cloth. Keep aside in a cool, dark place to germinate. In summer it will germinate by the evening, but in winter you will need to keep it in a warm place and the seeds will germinate by the morning. Once the little sprouts emerge, the bulk will increase. Have with half a cup of fresh bitter gourd juice and a teaspoon of honey once a day. The seeds should be germinated every day so that there is a stock of fresh, black gram sprouts daily. This recipe is especially beneficial for those who have mild diabetes. The milk from sprouted, ground black gram dal, and also that of plain Bengal gram sprouts, potentiates the action of naturally available insulin.

- Ayurveda recommends the use of saffron in a number of kidney ailments. Take a pinch of saffron dissolved in a teaspoon of milk, add half a teaspoon of honey, and have it once a day.

- A herbal tea made with a teaspoon of dried Indian gooseberry powder and a teaspoon of sandalwood paste, taken once a day, is beneficial for persons with

---

FRESH JUICE EXTRACTED FROM THE OUTER LEAVES OF A FULL-GROWN CABBAGE IS GOOD FOR OBESITY AS WELL AS DIABETES. IT CUTS DOWN ON THE TOTAL INSULIN REQUIREMENT. IN SOME WAY IT REGULATES THE PANCREAS, THYROID AND ADRENAL FUNCTIONS.

a *pitha* constitution, but not for sedentary, laid-back *kapha* types.

■ Curry leaf is an essential ingredient in the South Indian diet. It is used to flavour dals, *rasam*, *sambar*, chutney and pickles. Eating 10-15 fresh leaves in the morning aids digestion and maintains the correct sugar level. In fact, it has a hypoglycemic or blood sugar-lowering action.

■ Similarly, fresh, tender leaf buds from the mango and neem tree, a teaspoon of each, crushed or made into a coarse paste, taken once a day, has a cleansing action on the digestive system; certain essential substances in these balance the inner environment, getting rid of toxins.

■ Dried, tender mango buds, or dried mango flowers (powdered), to which an equal amount of dried jambul-seed powder is added, can be stored. Take a tablespoonful of this every morning with hot water.

■ Have half a teaspoon of fine cummin seed powder twice a day with water.

■ Half a teaspoon of finely ground dry ginger powder and dried fennel powder, with a little honey, made into a paste, had thrice a day, is good for overall kidney function.

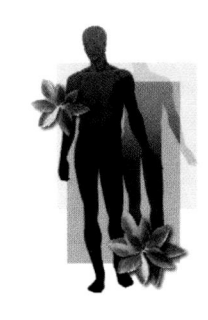

■ Eating figs is considered healthy – its pulp is nourishing and it has a laxative action. A little-known fact is that the fig seed, with the pulp removed, washed, dried and taken whole or as a powder—a teaspoon of the seed powder with a teaspoon of honey once a day—regularises blood sugar levels. Everything is utilised in nature, and so the seed too has its function.

■ The dried bark of the banyan tree has a decided role in lowering blood sugar. Some vital constituents have been known to lower fasting blood sugar levels as well as potentiate action on available insulin. A decoction made from dried bark powder—a tablespoon in two cups of water, boiled, reduced to half a cup, cooled, filtered and drunk once a day, is beneficial. To make an infusion, soak two tablespoons of dried powdered bark in a glass of hot water. Drink the filtrate next morning. The active anti-diabetic factor is a leucocyanidin derivative.

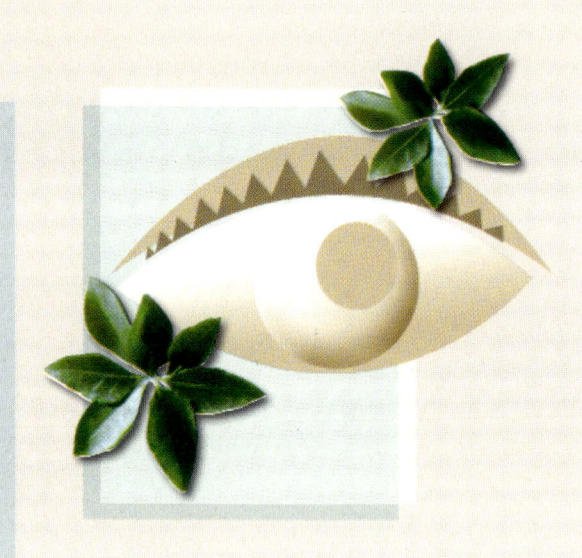

Our eyes are our windows to the world. Without them we would be trapped forever in darkness, devoid of light and colour. Hence, all eye problems, whether they are infections, degenerative problems or eye injuries, should receive urgent remedial care.

■ DISORDERS OF THE EYES

Eyes are a wonderful gift of nature, a vital organ in the human body, which makes us aware of the physical world, visually, to appreciate it in its totality. The eyes are delicate organs, embryologically an extension of the brain. They are lodged securely in two bony sockets in front of the skull, which protects them at all times. And yet, we have health problems related to the eyes.

Causes and symptoms

Pain, irritation, redness and watering of the eyes are symptoms common to many afflictions of the eyes. The commonest causes are dust, pollen and pollution. Tiredness of eyes due to poor diet, incorrect lighting while reading, extended periods of watching TV or video, working on the computer at an incorrect distance, being out in the sun for too long, or allergy to eye make-up, are the other causes. The more disturbing ones are bacterial or viral infections, reactions to certain systemic drugs, degenerative disorders, metabolic disorders, or refractive error. For all these problems, specific allopathic treatment is needed. However, some of these complementary remedies will aid in complete healing.

CONJUNCTIVITIS

This is a condition when the delicate membrane which lines the eyelids and covers the eyeballs is inflamed. It can be acute or chronic.

Causes and symptoms

The acute form of conjunctivitis is highly contagious and is caused by an infection. Conjunctivitis can also be the result of an allergy to airborne allergens such as pollen, dust, spores, animal hair, or certain plants. Congestion, redness and irritation characterise this condition. If the cause is dust, there is temporary irritation and a watery discharge. Allergy causes a marked redness in the eyes and profuse watering. There is immense discomfort and grittiness, as if there is

MUSTARD

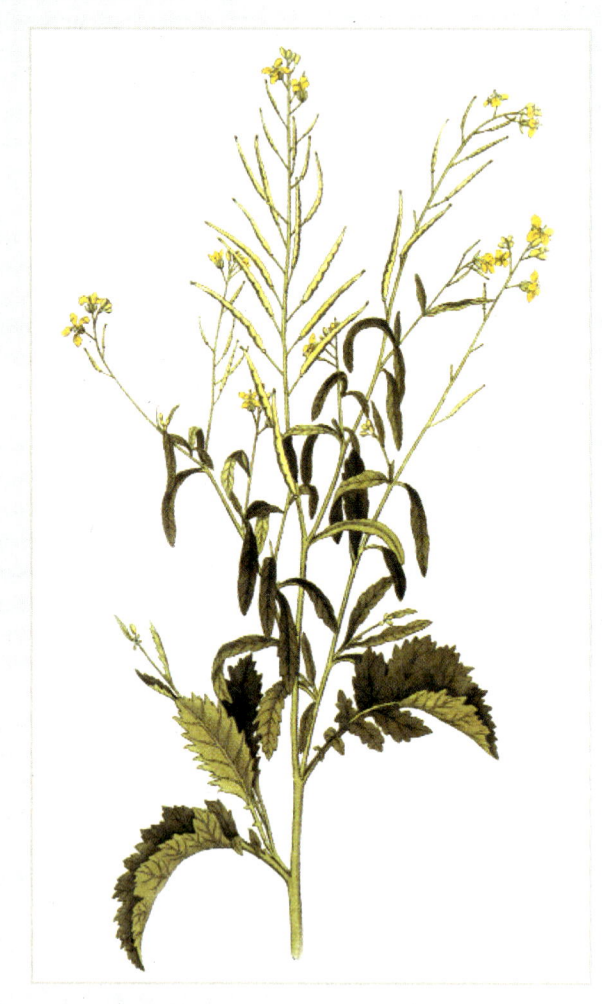

Botanical name: *Brassica alba*

Description and uses: The mustard plant has slender pods and beautiful yellow flowers.

Mustard seeds are used as a condiment and for medicinal purposes in paste and powder form. The oil extracted from them also has numerous uses, and is an important ingredient in many herbal remedies. Mustard is a stimulant, diuretic and emetic, and also used as a poultice in pneumonia, bronchitis and other diseases of the respiratory system. It is efficacious in the alleviation of neuralgia and other pains, and also massages and local applications. The application of mustard oil benefits rheumatism. The seed is useful in all its forms for treatment related to the head, conjunctivitis, disorders of the nose, gingivitis, toothache, throat problems, earache, muscle sprains and strains, chilblains, boils and other skin problems.

sand in the eyes. There is also marked photophobia. The person is not able to keep his eyes open or look at light. If the discharge is thick and pus-like, it is most likely a bacterial infection. Serious discharge points to a viral cause. In viral infections, there are velvet-like papillary projections or follicles on the under-surface of the eyelids.

Untreated conjunctivitis can cause inversion of the eyelid, corneal ulceration leading to perforation, and inflammation of all parts of the eyeball—the cornea is the transparent layer covering the front of the eye.

Remedies

Use herbal remedies at the first signs of discomfort, i.e., pain, redness or watering.

■ Boil a teaspoon of turmeric in two cups of water. Reduce it to one cup. Cool. Strain 4-5 times through a fine muslin. This extract can be used as an eye drop—a drop in the infected eye 3-4 times a day.

■ Boil a teaspoon of coriander seeds with a cupful of water for a while, like a herbal tea preparation. Use this to wash the eyes 3-4 times a day.

■ Strain fresh coriander-leaf juice 3-4 times through thin muslin. A drop of the strained juice should be put in each eye.

■ Boil a handful of acacia leaves in two cups of water. Make a decoction and use as a compress on the eyelids. It reduces swelling and pain.

■ Take a cup of water. Dissolve 2-3 granules of alum in it. Use as an eyewash.

■ Guava leaves, warmed and placed on a warm damp cloth, and then used as a compress, reduce the redness, pain and swelling.

■ Filter the fresh juice of a pomegranate. Put a drop in each inflamed eye for 1-3 days. It reduces the redness and burning sensation. If juice is not available, then a decoction can be made from the pounded dry peel of the fruit.

■ Boil, filter and wash eyes with a glass of water to which a teaspoon of turmeric has been added, 3-4 times a day. This has an antiseptic action.

■ Slit an aloe leaf lengthwise (the leaves are thick). Place the pulpy side on the sore eye. It reduces itchiness in inflamed and sore eyes.

■ A teaspoon of dried *emblica*

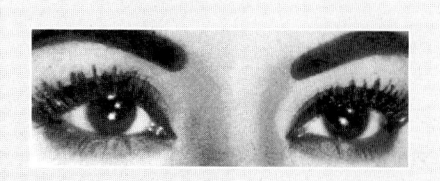

In rural areas, till quite recently (before the advent of eyeliner and mascara in India), an excellent eyeliner, *kajal*, was made at home. Fresh neem-leaf paste was applied to a cotton wick and dried. It was then soaked in mustard oil, to which a pinch of camphor was added. Then this was burnt to ashes. The residue was used as eyeliner or *kajal*. It caused initial smarting and watering of the eyes, but ensured that no infections occurred. The watering took care of any dust or foreign particles by washing them away. *Kajal* should only be used once a day. Too much 'cleansing' of normal eyes would defeat the purpose.

officinalis powder, boiled with a glass of water, is used as an eyewash to soothe sore eyes.

- A grated raw potato, used as a poultice, reduces swelling in inflamed eyes.

- Another poultice is made by baking or grilling an apple. Mash it, wrap it in a damp cloth, and while it is still very warm, but not enough to cause burns, use it as a poultice

- Take a small piece of turmeric, a pea-sized alum granule, and two tablespoons of fresh tamarind leaves. Grind them together to a paste with water. Place on a damp muslin cloth. Warm and use as a poultice

- Take a teaspoon each of holy basil and *bael*-leaf juice and a little milk. Cook till nearly charred black. Use as *kajal*.

- Mix about a teaspoon each of drumstick-seed oil, and a teaspoon of honey. Make a *kajal* and apply at bedtime. Drumstick seeds have certain antibiotic properties.

- Infusions made of coriander seeds or fennel seeds can be used as cold eyewashes too.

■ If there is only a sensation of burning, and not much redness or swelling, as when cutting pungent onions or going out in the hot sun, cool the eyes with a cold compress. Direct cold application of a little cream of cow's milk or fresh yoghurt will also soothe the eyes. The application should be cold.

■ Watering of the eyes: To a glassful of water, add a teaspoon of turmeric powder (made at home). Boil it for 10 minutes. Strain. Wash eyes with it.

STYE

A stye is a localised infection of one or more of the sebaceous glands in the eyelid. It has all the signs of inflammation, swelling, redness, pain, and heat or warmth, and occurs on the edge of the eyelid.

Cause and symptoms

These sebaceous glands lie just below the root of the eyelashes lining the eyelid edge, and their secretions keep the eyelid moist and lubricated. They are different from lachrymal or tear glands. Styes are extremely painful. One feels as though there is a a foreign body in the eye, and there is excessive watering and swelling of the eyelids. Looking at bright light hurts the eye. After about two days, when the swelling increases, a pus point forms in the indurated area. The abscess ruptures, releasing thick pus, and causes relief from the agonising pain.

Remedies

All the remedies—compresses or poultices for conjunctivitis—are beneficial for reducing the pain and swelling in a stye.

■ Fomenting with poultices of fresh steamed cabbage leaves, or bread soaked in hot milk, or grated raw potato, is very helpful and causes the abscess to rupture.

REFRACTIVE ERROR

We are able to see when light rays from an object enters the cornea, which is the transparent layer covering the front of the eye. The rays then pass through the lens, which lies behind the cornea, then through a fluid medium, and finally strike the nerve layer of the eyeball, called the retina. This is the innermost layer of the eyeball. This layer has specialised cells, which are sensitive to dim and bright light, and also to colour. The image of the object falls on the retina and is interpreted by the brain for us to visualise what it is. The whole mechanism involves the basic principles of physics, related to light, which travels in a straight line. When it travels from one medium to another it deviates from its straight path. This convergence or divergence affects the distance at which the object's image is formed. The curvature of the eyeball, in different planes, the muscles which move the eyeballs in different directions, the transparency of the lens, the state of the small muscles which contract or dilate the pupil of the eye, the fluid in the different chambers of the eye, and lastly, the state of the retinal cells, all play a part in the functioning of the eye and our vision.

Causes and symptoms

When refractive error is caused by the curvature of the eyeball, or the state of the lens, it is corrected by wearing prescribed spectacles and doing eye exercises.

Remedies

A remedy popular with many medical students of my generation:

Soak an almond in a cup of water at night. In the morning, peel and eat it with a cup of milk. It is rich in vitamin-A. On the second night, soak two almonds, and eat them the next morning. Add an almond every day for a week, till you are having seven almonds. The next night soak six almonds, and the next five, till at the end of the week you are again having only one almond. Eating these soaked almonds in an ascending and descending order is grandmother's prescription for good eyeright and healthy 'grey matter'. It also delays the onset of cataract. Almonds are highly nutritious and easily digestible proteins. Their brown skin is considered to be 'heat-producing' and also difficult to digest, and is hence discarded.

■ Eat plenty of carrots, red peppers, mangoes and melons. All fruits and vegetables in shades of yellow and orange, as well as green leafy vegetables, are rich in beta-carotene, the precursor of retinol.

■ Myopia or short-sightedness is benefited by the intake of a mixture of half a teaspoon of powdered liquorice root, half a teaspoon of ghee made from milk fat, and half a teaspoon of honey, thrice a day with half a cup of milk, before meals for 3-4 weeks.

Chinese medicine claims that liquorice has muscle-strengthening properties. Its beneficent action in myopia may be due to the strengthening of eyeball muscles and the ciliary muscles. Modern medicine, though, does not validate this claim. However, hypertensives need to be cautious regarding this remedy as it may cause retention of sodium and depletion of potassium in the body.

■ A cup of carrot juice and one-fourth of a cup of spinach juice taken twice a day is good for eyesight. Regular intake ensures that spectacles are never needed!

■ *Triphala churna*, made with Indian gooseberry (dried fruit pulp without seeds), *terminalia belerica* (the dried rind of the fruit), and *terminalia chebula* (the dried rind of the fruit), in equal measures by weight, is dried and powdered and then mixed together.

Practically all Indian households have these three ingredients in their homes. They are considered vital for healthy living. Half to one level teaspoon of this

---

IT IS SAFER TO GET YOUR VITAMIN REQUIREMENTS FROM FOOD RATHER THAN FROM TABLETS. AN EXCESS OF VITAMIN-A IS HARMFUL. BUT IF TAKEN IN NATURAL FOODS, IT IS JUST ENOUGH FOR US TO REMAIN IN GOOD HEALTH AND HAVE HEALTHY EYESIGHT.

RECENT STUDIES HAVE SHOWN THAT BETA-CAROTENE PROTECTS THE EYES FROM DAMAGE, WHICH OCCURS WHEN WORKING IN BRIGHT LIGHT, OR TOO MANY HOURS SPENT WORKING IN FRONT OF THE COMPUTER SCREEN. TWO OF THESE CAROTENOIDS ALSO PROTECT AGAINST AGE-RELATED DEGENERATIVE CHANGES. IN ANY DAMAGE TO TISSUE DUE TO ENVIRONMENTAL CAUSES, STRESS OR DEGENERATIVE DISORDERS, FREE RADIALS ARE LIBERATED FROM THE DAMAGED TISSUE. THESE ARE HARMFUL AND FURTHER DAMAGE HEALTHY TISSUE. BETA-CAROTENES NEUTRALISE FREE RADICALS AND PROTECT TISSUE.

mixture, taken daily, eliminates most disorders caused by a maladjustment of *kapha, pitta and vatta*— the ayurvedic descriptions of different types of body constitutions. It is recommended that for eye problems *triphala churna* should be taken with fresh ghee made from cow's milk or honey. Normally, for *vatta* constitutions, ghee is added, for *pitta*, milk, and for *kapha*, honey. In summers, it should be taken along with the evening meal, in winter after the meal, and during the monsoons with a pinch of rock salt after meals.

GLAUCOMA

There is fluid in front of and behind the lens of the eyes. This is maintained at an optimum pressure predetermined by nature.

Causes and symptoms

In glaucoma, fluid pressure builds up inside the eye and damages the delicate tissues of the eyes. This causes a throbbing headache and pain in and above the eyes. A person thinks he or she is seeing coloured rings around lights and lighted objects, and there is a gradual loss of peripheral vision.

Glaucoma can occur due to a congenital cause, but it is often a disease of the middle-aged and the elderly, striking people around 40 years of age and above. It often runs in families. Scientifically, it has been linked to a deficiency of vitamin-B (thiamine), vitamin-C and vitamin-A.

Remedy

If the symptoms given above are present, do not try home remedies, but get an eye check-up done by an ophthalmologist. Glaucoma can cause total loss of vision if it is not treated in time.

■ A diet rich in green leafy vegetables and foods which are yellow or orange-coloured will ensure the right vitamin intake.

> ## FOREIGN BODY IN THE EYE, OR INJURY TO THE EYE
>
> IF THERE IS ANY DUST OR POLLEN IN THE EYE, WASH IT WITH CLEAN WATER. DO NOT ATTEMPT REMOVING ANYTHING FROM THE EYE ON YOUR OWN. IF THIS FAILS TO BRING RELIEF, CONSULT AN OPHTHALMOLOGIST. ANY INJURY TO THE EYE MUST, REPEAT, MUST, BE SEEN TO BY A DOCTOR.

CATARACT

The lens of the eyes are transparent, flexible and made of crystalline tissue.

Causes and symptoms

Gradual clouding of the lens, with loss of transparency and gradually deteriorating vision, is called the 'the coming on of cataract' or cataract formation. This normally occurs in an aging person. However, some newborns can be born with it, or it can be acquired at a young age due to metabolic disorders, e.g., diabetes or galactose metabolic disorders.

Remedies

■ A diet rich in vitamin-B, especially riboflavin, which is found in milk, and vitamin-A, in green leafy vegetables, etc., delay the onset of cataract. Wholegrain cereals and yeast extract added to the diet are beneficial.

■ Fresh wheatgrass juice taken daily, and also used as eye drops once a day, is efficacious. It should be consumed immediately after extraction and should be about one-third of a cup, sipped slowly so that the saliva mixes with it. If you find it unpalatable, flavour it with fresh grape juice or a little honey. Wheatgrass juice protects cell membrane and maintains its transparency.

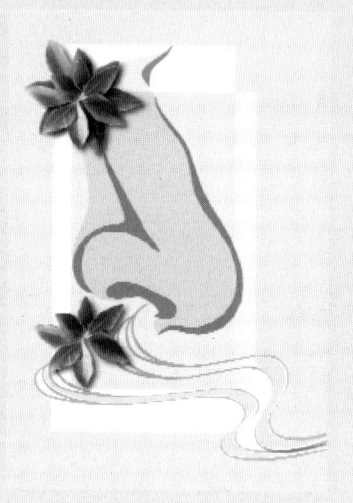

We breathe through our noses mainly—inhale oxygen and exhale carbon dioxide and other waste gases. Any problem with the nose disrupts healthy breathing. Colds, nosebleeds, or a foreign body in the nose, therefore, need immediate attention.

■ DISORDERS OF THE NOSE

Just as the eyes are a gift from nature, to make us visually aware of the physical world in its totality, the nose is the gateway to our breathing apparatus—the respiratory system. We inhale fresh air—life-giving and sustaining—through our noses and mouths. The *prana* enters the system via the nose, and any problem there disrupts good, healthy breathing.

Causes and symptoms

The harbinger of most problems related to the respiratory system is a cold, a running nose, sneezing, etc. Modern medicine suggests that these symptoms may just be the onset of a mild seasonal infection, or an allergy such as hay fever, but may also signify the prodomal symptoms of a severe viral infection, influenza, or may result in inflammation of the sinuses in the facial bones—sinusitis.

Ayurveda, however, attributes this to an imbalance in eating habits, especially in a diet which comprises mainly of refined food—bread, milk, cheese, salt, sugar, etc. These increase the *kapha dosas*, whereby a person is extremely susceptible to variations in environmental temperature, exposure to draughts, etc., and this results in a running nose, phlegm, sneezing, etc.

Apparently headaches, loss of appetite, constipation, bodyaches, tiredness are all connected to a cold. This often involves the entire respiratory passage, sometimes resulting in the life-threatening diseases pneumonia.

Remedies

■ A tried and tested remedy, taken at the onset of a cold in most Indian homes, is a glass of hot milk with a teaspoon of turmeric powder, and a teaspoon of jaggery or sugar, twice a day.

■ Boil a teaspoon of turmeric powder and one-fourth of a teaspoon of omum in three cups of water. Make a decoction. Take a teaspoon of this decoction with a teaspoon of honey 2-3 times a day.

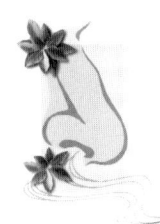

Note: *Fresh turmeric, in its raw state, acquired from the earth as a rhizome, is used in herbal dyes. However, for it to be edible, it is boiled and dried and sold in the market either whole or powdered. Turmeric has antiseptic properties. In its raw state, it has a volatile oil which has cholesterol-lowering properties.*

- Nasal congestion and a stuffy nose are often relieved by inhaling steam from a pan more than half full of boiling water, to which a tablespoon of powdered omum seeds have been added.

- Oral intake of omum or inhalation is beneficial in colds which occur in winter. Avoid omum for a common cold at the beginning of summer, as it is a 'hot' substance.

- Or use a tablespoon of powdered omum wrapped in a fine muslin handkerchief, warmed against a hot iron vessel, for fomentation on the nose or chest.

- Take a dried peepul leaf, put powdered omum on it. Roll it like a cigarette and smoke or inhale it. This clears the respiratory passages.

- Grind together and extract the juice of a medium-sized betel leaf, 4-5 holy basil leaves and a half-inch piece of ginger. Add honey to taste and have about half a tablespoon 2-3 times a day.

- For those who like a drink, especially on a winter evening, and are feeling low due to a cold, this is just the remedy to raise their spirits! However, limit yourself to just one drink. Mix in a glass of hot water the juice of one lemon, a teaspoon of honey and two tablespoons of brandy, and drink it.

- Mix together a teaspoon of fresh or dried holy basil leaves, a pinch each of clove powder and cinnamon powder. Boil a cup of water. Add the mixture to it, with honey to taste. Drink it.

- A summer cold, which persists for a long time and becomes sinusitis (inflammation of the sinuses, causing a headache), with a thick discharge from the nose, responds well to a mixture of a teaspoon of ground black pepper, half a cup of fresh curd, and two teaspoons of jaggery powder. This should be taken twice a day for some time—a week or 10 days.

- Boil in a cup of water a teaspoon each of liquorice and cinnamon powders, and a tablespoon of fresh ginger paste, or a teaspoon of dried ginger powder, for 5-8 minutes. Filter. A refreshing, stimulating

> If you have eucalyptus growing nearby, crush a handful of tender leaves and boil them in a litre of water. Take inhalations 3-4 times a day. The steam and essential oils in the leaves are wonderfully soothing and relieve the congestion in the entire respiratory tract. Sage, mint or thyme leaves can also be used.
>
> A lesser-known remedy is to prepare a foot bath with 4-6 tablespoons of ground mustard seeds, boiled in a litre of water. Make a decoction. Filter, add the filtrate to a basinful of hot water, and soak your feet in it for 10-15 minutes. Keep your feet soaked till the water is of room temperature. This acts as a counter irritant. It stimulates the nerve endings in the feet and improves circulation. However, mustard seeds or oil contain irritant factors and can cause irritation of the skin. So be careful while using them. Not for people with sensitive skin!

herbal tea! Drink it with a teaspoon of honey.

- Make a gruel with two tablespoons of broken wheat, in which the wheat husk has not been removed, and 8-10 peppercorns. Add salt to taste and boil till soft. Mash, strain and have twice a day.

- For those who suffer from perpetual colds throughout the year, a decoction made with a tablespoon of crushed holy basil leaves, 2-3 cloves of garlic and five peppercorns, ground together and boiled with water, is an efficacious remedy. Have twice a day for a week.

- Tamarind tea: To make tamarind tea, make tamarind pulp by soaking a tablespoon of dried tamarind in a cup of water. Boil and leave aside. When it cools, mash, remove seeds and strain. Sweeten with honey, jaggery or sugar, and have 2-3 times a day.

- Onion soup: To make onion soup, cut 2-3 large onions in slices; 2-3 cloves of garlic, crushed or finely chopped; a few dried omum leaves, 1-2 sage leaves, and a bay leaf; some vegetable or chicken stock; the juice of half a lime. Fry the onions and garlic till they are light brown in colour. Add the crushed herbs and cook for another 2-3 minutes. Add 4-5 cups of stock and cook on a low fire for 30-40 minutes, stirring off and on. Strain, add salt and pepper to taste, and have the soup twice a day.

- Mix together half a tablespoon of powdered omum and one-fourth of a teaspoon of rock salt, and gulp it down with warm water. In the case of persistent colds, this mixture, taken once or twice a week, aids the digestion. According to ayurvedic philosophy, impaired digestion causes susceptibility to repeated colds, coughs and chest infections. If the digestion process is set right, the functions of the entire body are re-balanced.

- Mix a teaspoon of jaggery powder with a pinch of asafoetida and one-fourth of a teaspoon of black pepper powder, and have with warm water twice a day. This is especially helpful for people who are prone to indigestion with flatulence and a persistent cold.

- Boil two heaped tablespoons of freshly ground coriander seeds with two glasses of water, and make a decoction till just half a glass of water is left. Add *misri*—lump sugar. The resultant mixture will be of the consistency of chutney or sauce. Take one-fourth of a teaspoon twice or thrice a day for 2-4 weeks. It helps to clear the respiratory passages of phlegm, and should be placed on the tongue and savoured.

- A variation of the previous remedy is to mix finely ground coriander seeds with an equal quantity of pounded jaggery, and half to one teaspoon should be taken 3-4 times a day.

- To pre-empt a winter cold, a level teaspoon of dried ground ginger with an equal quantity of jaggery, ground together, should be taken thrice a day.

- A teaspoon of fresh ginger juice with a teaspoon of honey, taken twice a day, aborts an incipient cold. You can add the juice of a few holy basil leaves to this, in case you feel there is a fever coming on.

NOSEBLEEDS

Nosebleeds are sometimes the aftermath of a blow on the nose in a fistfight between 'unequals', or it may be due to other reasons.

Causes and symptoms

Blood vessels that supply the nasal mucosa are very delicate. Blowing one's nose hard or removing a scab from the nostril can cause a nosebleed. Unprovoked bleeding from the nose may be a sign of undiagnosed hypertension. Sometimes a head injury may show no apparent external symptoms except a nosebleed. Do not treat it at home—rush to the doctor. It may be the first indication of something seriously amiss. Being outdoors during a particularly hot summer day may also cause a nosebleed.

Remedies

■ Make the patient sit down and pinch his or her nose at the junction of the bony and soft parts, just at the edge of the sides of the bony prominence. Plug the bleeding nostril with a cottonwool swab.

■ Grind fresh coriander leaves and put one or two drops of its juice into the nostril. This will cause the bleeding to stop.

■ Mango flowers are another effective remedy. The juice has an antistyptic action.

FOREIGN ARTICLE IN THE NOSE

Children are notorious for pushing pebbles or small buttons up their noses. Blowing the nose hard or inducing a sneeze often pops the offending article out. Sniff ammonia, pungent onion juice or pepper, and a sneeze will follow, dislodging the foreign article.

INJURY TO THE NOSE

Administer first-aid in minor injuries, like checking an obvious external nosebleed. For more serious complaints, see a doctor.

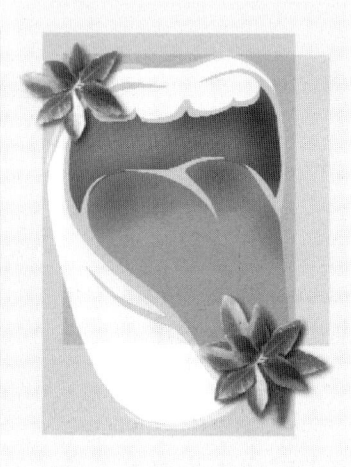

As we eat and drink with our mouths, the importance of taking adequate care of our teeth, and gums, and keeping the mucus membranes healthy, cannot be overemphasised. Prevention rather than cure should be the motto as far as mouth care is concerned.

MOUTH PROBLEMS

The mouth is the entrance to our gastrointestinal tract. All the food we eat goes thorough this portal. Its mucous membrane is subjected to various stimuli—hot tea, ice, ice cream, sour chutney, etc. It's a wonder it stays as smooth and soft as it is. The beginning of any problem in the body often starts as small, often neglected lesions in this area.

CHAPPED LIPS

Chapped lips are a very common problem and most people are unable to tackle it effectively.

Causes and symptoms

The vagaries of weather effect the lips. The advent of cold winter winds brings in its wake chapped lips. Summer takes its toll for those who sunbathe or swim. One of the symptoms of a high temperature is dry chapped lips.

Remedies

- The application of coconut oil or ghee on dry chapped lips is a common practice in middle-class Indian homes.

- A lesser-known remedy is to put a little ghee or butter into the navel at night before going to sleep. How this works is anyone's guess, but work it does! It is a tried and tested remedy.

- Heat a teaspoonful of ghee and add a pinch of salt to it. Apply this as a lip salve.

- Take some fresh cream of just boiled milk. Add a few drops of fresh lime juice to it. Mix and gently massage on the lips. Wipe off or just dab with a soft tissue.

- Glycerine and fresh lime juice can be mixed in equal proportions and kept in a bottle. This can be applied on the face and lips in winter after a hot-water bath.

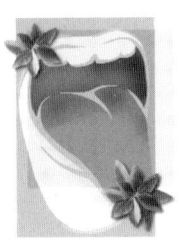

SORE MOUTH

Ulcers in the mouth/ apthous ulcers / cold sores or herpes simplex: These are lesions in the mucus membrane of the mouth.

Causes and symptoms

Apthous ulcers or ulcers in the mouth are small white spots on the inside of the cheek, the inner surface of the lips, sides of the tongue, on or below the tongue, palate, or anywhere on the mucus membrane of the mouth. Initially they are white, but sometimes small ones occur close together, coalase and appear like a large red ulcer with a grayish base. These are extremely painful.

These ulcers may be caused by certain deficiencies in the diet, e.g., of the B-complex vitamins. They could also be due to any illness for which antibiotics are being taken. Antibiotics wash away the normal flora present in our intestinal tract, which produces the required enzymes which act on the B-complex present in the ingredients in our diet. At times, nervous tension/ stress results in a tense, clamped jaw, or the person bites the inside of the mouth, injuring the mucosa, which results in an ulcer. Certain foods, especially spices, chillies, and some food additives, are often other culprits.

Herpes simplex, a viral infection, also results in cold sores which begin as small white clusters of sores on the inside of the lip. They cause intense pain and salivation, are an angry red in colour, and they coalesce to form a desquamating upper crust. This infection is often precipitated by a debilitated, physically run-down condition—the aftermath of some other illness. Chronic constipation and an upset digestion are also causes of mouth ulcers.

Remedies

These remedies soothe and relieve pain:

■ Gargling with hot water, or holding hot water in the mouth on the area of the ulcer, helps to relieve the pain. This should be done 3-4 times a day.

■ Boil some zyziphus leaves in water to make a strong herbal tea, and use this to gargle 3-4 times a day.

■ Make a light decoction of guava leaves and gargle with it 3-4 times a day.

■ Add half a teaspoon of turmeric and

one-fourth of a teaspoon of rock salt in a glass of hot water. Gargle with it thrice a day.

- A teaspoon of roasted, pounded *neem* bark mixed with half a teaspoon of catechu, and this powder applied on an ulcer, causes intense salivation. This should be spat out, and then the person should gargle with warm water 3-4 times a day.

- Applying boro-glycerine thrice a day causes intense salivation followed by relief.

- Catechu can also be made into a powder, and then into a thick paste with water. Apply this on the ulcers.

- To half a teaspoon of fine, powdered small cardamoms, add half a teaspoon of roasted, powdered alum. Take a pinch of the mixture, place it on the ulcer and close the mouth. There will be intense salivation. Keep it in the mouth for 30 seconds and then spit it out. Gargle with warm water and repeat the whole process once again. Do this 2-3 times a day.

- Jasmine, which grows well in hilly areas, has varied properties, one of which is to soothe pain and heal chronic skin

Mode of action: Turmeric is an antiseptic, jambul leaves and Spanish jasmine leaves have a soothing demulcent action, while all the other ingredients cited in the remedies given above have an astringent action. They draw the exudate out from the base of the swelling, thereby relieving the pain caused by the pressure exerted by the fluid on the tiny nerve endings. Pressure is perceived as pain by the interpreting mechanism of the brain. The exudate and excess salivation also washes out the inflammatory debris, hastening normal healing of the mucosa. Being green, these ingredients have vitamin-C, beta-carotene and other trace elements, which all contribute to the repair of damaged tissue.

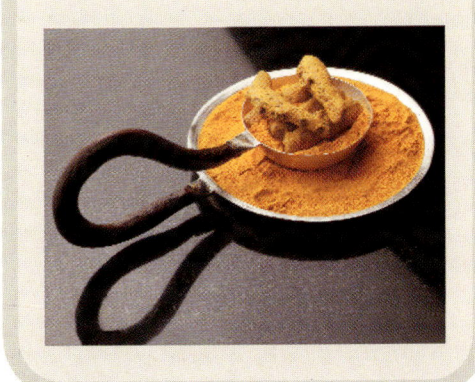

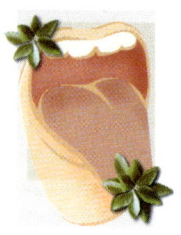

inflammation / ulcers of the mucous membrane.

- Liquorice also has anti-inflammatory properties akin to corticosteroids.

- *Terminalia chebula* is a dried fruit commonly found in Indian kitchens, though not exactly used as a spice or condiment. It has astringent and laxative properties. All Indian systems of medicine emphasise the importance of a clear stomach/bowels as a criterion for good health. The following is an age-old household remedy for a healthy lifestyle.

Take equal quantities of *terminalia chebula*, jasmine, liquorice and barberry leaves. Dry them in the shade, grind them to a fine powder, mix, sieve and store in a dry bottle. For an ulcer in the mouth, take a large pinch of the mixture, add a few drops of honey to make a smooth paste, and apply on it. Salivation will take place, but even if the mixture is swallowed, it is not harmful. Apply thrice a day. It will soothe the pain, reduce the inflammation, and also cure heartburn, dyspepsia and indigestion, which are often the cause of these ulcers.

- Chew fresh carrot leaves and then wash it out with water. It prevents putrefaction of the slough at the base of the mouth ulcers.

- Make a cut in the thick stem of a banyan tree. A drop of the sap added to a drop of honey, and applied on the ulcer, heals it. Apply 2-3 times a day.

- A herbal tea made with a few crushed henna leaves added to a cup of lukewarm water, and then used as a gargle, soothes the ulcerated surface.

- A decoction of rose petals, with a dash of lime, used as a gargle, is also soothing when done 3-4 times a day.

- Take a handful of fresh, tender tamarind leaves. Make an infusion with a glass of hot water. It has antimicrobial properties, and its mildly acidic taste clears the loss of taste and unclean feeling in the mouth.

SORE GUMS / BLEEDING GUMS—GINGIVITIS

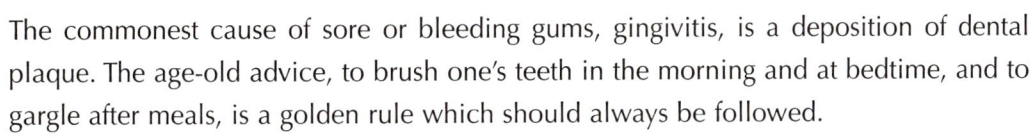

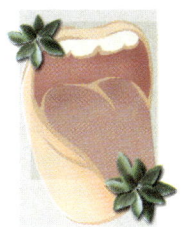

The commonest cause of sore or bleeding gums, gingivitis, is a deposition of dental plaque. The age-old advice, to brush one's teeth in the morning and at bedtime, and to gargle after meals, is a golden rule which should always be followed.

Causes and symptoms

When you eat anything, the teeth masticate the food before you swallow it. Some pieces may get lodged in the small crevices or at the base of the teeth. If these are not got rid of by brushing the teeth or gargling after meals, they keep collecting and harden to form plaques. They soften the junction of the teeth with the gum. This loosened area attracts bacteria and other micro-organisms, leading to mild, moderate or severe inflammation. This causes pain and sometimes even bleeding gums while brushing teeth. Bad breath, loose teeth, cavities in the teeth, are all associated with this problem. Sweets and carbohydrate-rich food aggravate it.

Vitamin deficiency, anaemia, allergic disorders, drug reactions, certain blood dyscrasis are other causes.

Remedies

■ Take a tablespoon of mustard oil and add a teaspoon of common salt to it. Wash your hands well. With the forefinger take a small amount of this mixture and massage the gums gently in upward, downward and circular strokes. Do this for 30 seconds and then gargle with warm water. Do this 2-3 times a day.

■ Take half a teaspoonful of omum. Grind it to a fine powder and add a few drops of mustard oil to it. Now use this to massage the gums. Gargle with warm water. Repeat at least twice a day.

■ Use a herbal tea made with henna leaves as a mouthwash.

■ The bark of acacia has astringent properties. Make a decoction, dilute and use it as a gargle thrice a day. It is very refreshing and leaves a sweet taste in the mouth.

■ Burn alum in a non-stick pan. Powder the burnt mass. Use a pinch of this as a tooth powder for gum massage. Gargle with plain water. Do this once or twice a day. It reduces spongy gums and heals toothache. Alum is an astringent.

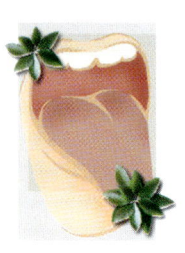

- Take a teaspoon of castor oil. Add a large pinch of powdered camphor to it. Mix and gently massage the gum with it. Rinse mouth with warm water.

- To prepare a soothing mouthwash for sore gums, boil 10-15 fresh eucalyptus leaves in a litre of water. Simmer for five minutes, then switch off heat. Cover and keep aside. Strain and add 2-3 drops of clove oil. If you do not have clove oil, add the powder of 6-7 finely ground cloves and bring the mixture to the boil again. Filter, cool and use as a mouthwash after every meal. This can be stored in the refrigerator for a few days

- Soft neem or acacia twigs should be used as tooth brushes. Chew on the twig till it softens and splits. This takes about five minutes. Then spit out the fragments and gargle. It is a disinfectant, and excellent for gum massage and mastication.

TOOTHACHE

The agony of a toothache can never be forgotten by anyone who has suffered from it. In this case, as in many others, prevention is better than cure.

Causes and symptoms

Tooth decay due to bad oro-dental hygiene or excessive intake of junk food, candy, soft aerated drinks, cakes and pastries, etc, will lead to the erosion of the enamel of the teeth, and this ultimately results in a toothache. A toothache can be mild, only occurring when eating something hot or cold, or it can be sharp, shooting, throbbing—this depends on the extent to which the nerve is exposed and is being irritated.

Remedies

- All the remedies given for gum massage will afford some relief for toothache. However, clove oil is specific for this problem. One may not have clove oil at home. In that case, powder some cloves very fine and make a strong decoction (literally a concentrate). Soak a cottonwool swab in this, place it on the hurting tooth, and very gently clamp your jaws tight. The medicament will reach the injured surface and soothe the pain.

CLOVES

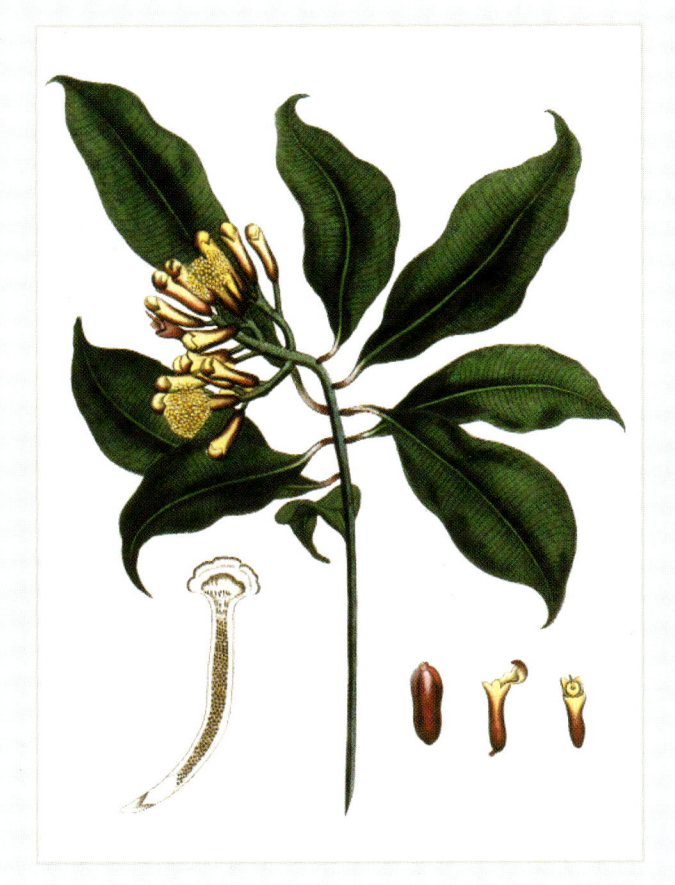

Botanical name: *Eugenia aromatica*

Description and uses: The clove tree is small and an evergreen. Its flowers grow in bunches at the end of the branches. The cloves used in cooking and for therapeutic uses are the dried flower buds of the tree, which are pungent and aromatic. They contain a large amount of essential oil, which is used for medicinal purposes. Good quality cloves are fat, oily and dark brown in colour. Clove powder and oil are very effective in treating fever, problems related to the head, nausea, hypertension, disorders of the nose, sore gums, toothache, earache, chest pain, coughs, digestive problems, diarrhoea, cholera, intestinal worms, arthritis, backache, blisters, boils, burns, sexual debility and morning sickness in pregnancy.

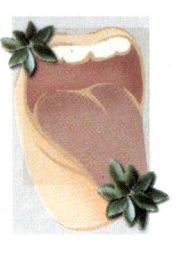

- Take a spoonful of banyan-tree (stem) sap. Mix it with honey, apply on the gums and leave it for 2-3 minutes. Then gargle. Do this twice a day.

- A spoonful of fresh onion juice, made from spring onions, old white onions, or onion flowers, is beneficial. However, a mixture made from fresh onions and onion flowers has more medicinal value. The fresh onions and the extract from the flowers are rich in sulphur compounds, which are bactericidal. Dip a swab of cottonwool in the fresh juice, and then plug the 'complaining' tooth with it. It is a little pungent and smelly, but will disinfect the inflamed tooth. Gargle with warm water.

- For those who have access to cashew trees. Chew 1-2 cashew leaves and let the juice remain in the mouth for 2-3 minutes.

TOOTH POWDERS

- Dried mint leaves can be ground fine and used as a tooth powder
- Grind a spoonful of rock salt, cummin seeds and black pepper to a fine powder.
- Finely powder, seperately, dry ginger, cloves, black pepper, betel-nuts and rock salt. Take equal measures of each, mix and bottle. Use half a teaspoonful as a tooth powder daily.
- Take a cupful of the bark of the peepul tree. Dry, pound and powder. Use half a teaspoonful to massage gums and teeth. Do not swallow. Gargle with hot and cold water alternately, 2-3 times, till the mouth feels clean. Once a day is enough.
- Mix equal amounts of finely powdered black pepper and salt. Use a pinch of this for gum massage and as a tooth powder. Gargle with lukewarm water. This is more of a preventive measure. For caries or cavities in the teeth, include an equal amount of powdered cloves. This will hurt a little initially, but after gargling there will be alleviation of pain.
- Do not discard almond shells. Collect a handful. Burn them to ashes and collect the burnt residue. Powder. Sieve and use as a tooth powder. This removes the yellowish deposit on the teeth and prevents tooth decay.
- Take a teaspoon each of dried powdered *terminalia chebula, terminalia belerica,* Indian gooseberry, black pepper, dried ginger, roasted alum and rock salt. Mix well and grind again. Use this as a tooth powder. Gargle well with warm water. Use twice a day.

Note: *If any of these ingredients seem too bitter, and you find it is difficult to use it as a tooth powder, a little arrowroot flour can be added to it, but it should not be stored with arrowroot mixed in it.*

Then spit it out and gargle with plain water. This relieves toothache, but does not cure the cause of the toothache.

- Crush 2-3 cloves and fry them in a spoonful of coconut oil. Remove them before they are burnt. Powder and apply them on the tooth.

- Boil half a teaspoon or a small piece of asafoetida in a cupful of water and gargle with it 2-3 times a day. Remove the piece, which will have softened, and place it in the cavity of the inflamed tooth. Keep it there for as long as you comfortably can, then remove it by gargling with warm water.

- Herbal tea made from fresh mango flowers acts as an astringent, soothes inflammation and relieves pain. Use as a mouthwash, but do not drink it as a tea.

- A tooth powder made of burnt mango leaves is beneficial in relieving toothache.

- Grate and powder nutmeg fine. Add one-fourth of a teaspoon of this powder to a teaspoon of warm mustard, sesame or coconut oil. Soak a cottonwool swab in this and place it on the hurting tooth. Keep it for a while and then remove it. Gargle with warm water. Nutmeg has a narcotic action, therefore this should be done only once a day for 1-2 days. Consult a dentist if there is no relief. Overdosage is dangerous as individual reactions vary and may lead to toxic effects—hallucination, restlessness, convulsions, etc.

- Powder fine green cardamom seeds, dried ginger and liquorice separately. Take a pinch of each, and make a paste with a few drops of honey. Apply it on the surface of the painful tooth. Leave it there for a few minutes and then wash it down with water.

- Fry a teaspoon of cloves in mustard/coconut/sesame oil. Remove the cloves from the oil and powder them. Apply it on the affected tooth. This is good as a gum massage too.

WISDOM TEETH

Any of the above remedies for toothache and spongy gums will give relief if used as a gum massage. But sometimes a wisdom tooth is impacted and will need expert surgical intervention by a dentist.

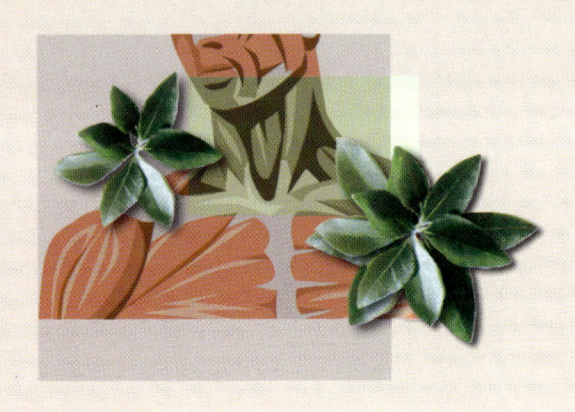

The throat is the gateway to the digestive and respiratory systems; the foodpipe and windpipe both originate there, and the voice box is situated there too. Therefore, any infection or problem in this area should not be neglected as it vitally affects breathing, swallowing, eating and speaking.

THROAT PROBLEMS

The throat is common to the digestive as well as the respiratory system. It lies at the beginning of the windpipe and the foodpipe. It also has the voice box where the windpipe commences. Hence, any infection or problem in the throat causes discomfort while eating, breathing, swallowing or speaking.

Causes and symptoms

On either side of the beginning of the windpipe lie two collections of tissues, not clearly discernable in a healthy state, called tonsils. Any infection causes them to increase in size, and they become painful—this is referred to as enlarged tonsils or tonsillitis. The root of this part of the throat is called the pharynx. The voice box is referred to as the larynx, the foodpipe is the oesophagus, and the windpipe is the trachea. These are standard medical terms.

Any infection in this area affects all these structures to a lesser or greater degree. Hence, the same herbal remedies relieve the symptoms of pain, swelling or discomfort. If the infection or area involved is specific, then one can have pharyngitis, tonsillitis laryngitis and trachiatis! The larynx can also become inflamed, leading to hoarseness of the voice, if one talks too loudly for too long.

Remedies

■ Gargle with warm water, with a pinch of salt in it, 3-4 times a day. Using too much salt, however, causes irritation and gagging, and often vomiting.

■ Boil in a cup of water, half a teaspoon each of finely powdered cinnamon and black pepper. Add honey and sip or drink it like tea, while it is warm—cinnamon has antiseptic properties. It also acts as an astringent, relieving any swelling caused by inflammation. Pepper has an active principle called pipperine. This gives it its characteristic pungent taste, and also imparts analgesic and anti-inflammatory qualities to it. To a certain extent, it mildly depresses the activities of the central nervous system.

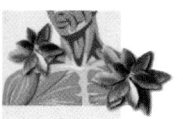

Whenever an infection occurs, there are 'macrophages', the body policemen, who run to engulf the invading organisms. They also produce nitro-oxide which prevents replication of the infecting virus. Pipperine enhances nitro-oxide production. Another molecule in the active principle enhances an antigen-specific protective response.

- Mix together and have a 'pinch' of powdered black pepper (11-12 seeds) and a level tablespoon of powdered lump sugar. Savour it as you would a toffee. Let the medicament trickle down your throat. The sweetness of candy will take away the pungency of the pepper. This mixture clears the throat.

- Boil and make an infusion with a cup of water and a teaspoonful of omum. Let it cool to a bearable temperature, but it should still be hot. Use this for gargling. A pinch of salt can be added to it. Or sip it like tea, with honey or sugar to taste.

- Mix a teaspoon of the finely powdered bark of a fig tree with a cupful of hot milk. Add sugar to taste. Drink this once a day for 4-5 days. It acts as an emollient and soothes inflamed, raw surfaces. However, it also has a mildly laxative action. So do not take too much of it.

- A teaspoon of fresh onion juice, flavoured with honey, mixed in a cup of warm water and sipped for a while once a day, relieves soreness in membranes subjected to loud talking, cheering or singing. This remedy has helped many a singer recover from the after-effects of a long vocal recital.

- A small piece of liquorice, kept in the mouth and sucked, or ground into fine powder and taken with a little sugar or honey and warm water, soothes a sore throat.

- Add a teaspoon of turmeric powder to two cups of water. Boil, strain and gargle with it.

- Crush and boil two garlic cloves in a cup of water. Strain and use for gargling.

- Tea made with holy basil is excellent for sore throats. Alternatively, chew 4-5 holy basil leaves for 10-15 minutes. Then swallow them with warm water or gargle. Do not let the residue of the leaves stick to your teeth. Their volatile oils have an anti-inflammatory action and heal and soothe an inflamed throat, but the green leaf deposit has traces of mercury which erodes tooth enamel. In any case, it is wise to gargle after every

PEPPER

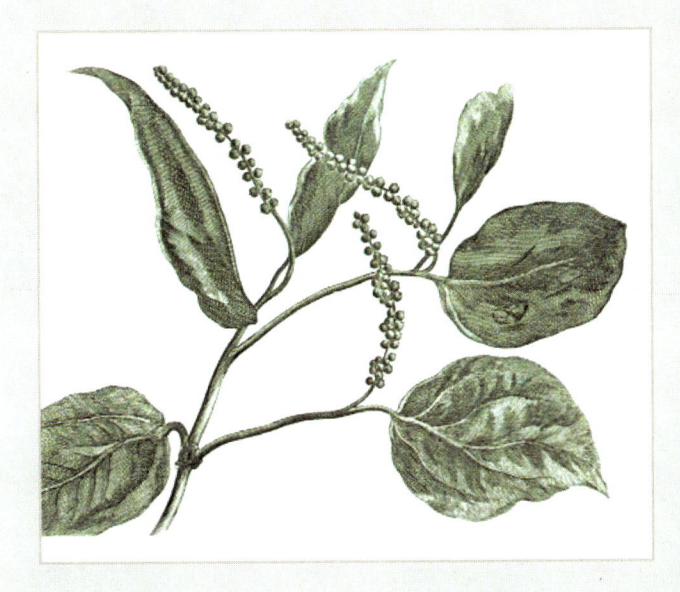

Botanical name:
Piper nigrum

Description and uses: The pepper plant is a perennial with a round, smooth, woody stem; the leaves are dark green and ovate; and the fruits globular red berries when ripe, with a coarsely wrinkled surface. The berries are collected as soon as they turn red, and are dried in the sun. Pepper has an aromatic odour and a pungent, bitterish taste. It has been greatly valued from time immemorial—so much so that it is said that Attila the Hun demanded 3000 lb of pepper in ransom for the city of Rome!

Apart from its other uses, pepper is highly efficacious as a herbal remedy. It has an active principle called pipperine, which gives it its pungent taste and analgesic and anti-inflammatory qualities. Whenever our bodies are under siege by an infection, the body policemen, the macrophages, rush to attack the invaders. They produce nitro-oxide, which prevents replication of the infecting virus. Pipperine enhances nitro-oxide production.

Pepper is a stimulant, a carminative, and is said to possess febrifuge properties. It is used to treat fevers, styes, disorders of the nose, throat problems, hoarseness, indigestion, constipation, cholera, jaundice, gallstones, loss of appetite, sexual debility, intestinal worms, diabetes and skin problems, and is an indispensable ingredient in herbal tooth powder

TURMERIC

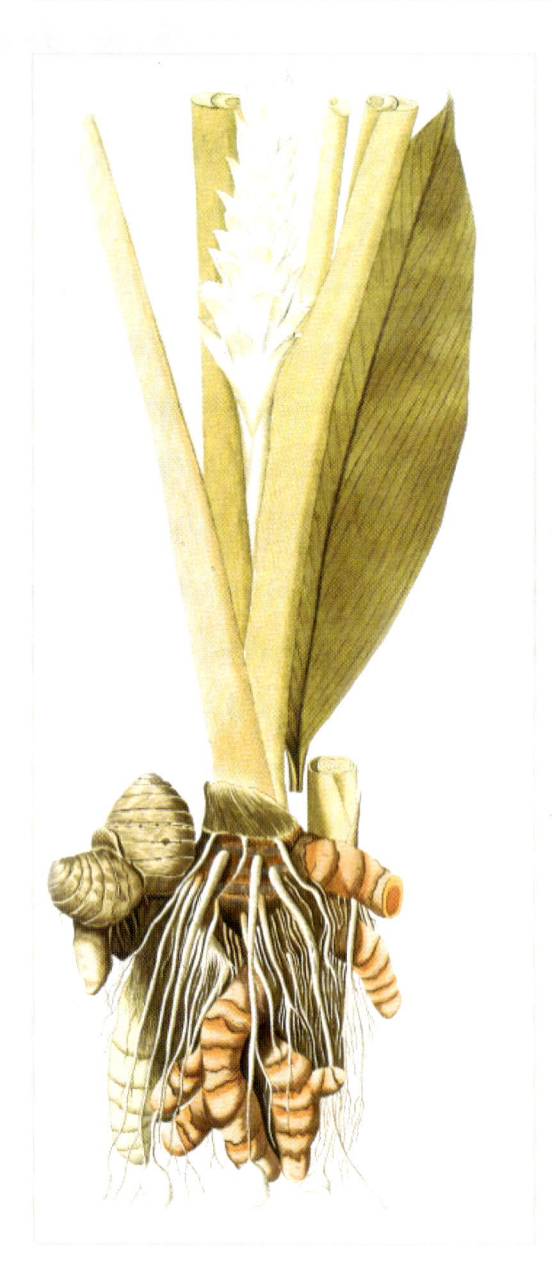

Botanical name: *Curcuma longa*

Description and uses: The turmeric plant is of the ginger family, yielding aromatic rhizomes which are used as a spice in curries, as dyes, and for medicinal purposes. It is yellow in colour and has an aromatic, slightly bitter taste—both in powder and paste form. Fresh and dried turmeric is used for multifarious ailments such as fever, anaemia, hypertension, conjunctivitis, disorders of the nose, a sore mouth, throat problems, chest pain, coughs, wheezing and other respiratory problems, digestive disorders, jaundice, diabetes, muscle strains and sprains, chapped lips, skin problems, wounds and sexual debility.

meal, or after eating anything. Protect your teeth!

- Chewing a half-inch-thin slice of fresh ginger, dipped in a little salt, also helps soothe sore throats.

- Depending on their availability, an infusion made with henna leaves (dried or fresh), or a handful of sage leaves, or fenugreek or tamarind leaves, used for gargling, is helpful in healing sore throats.

- Henna leaves have an astringent action. They also have antibacterial properties, whereas tamarind leaves have a soothing emollient action, in addition to their antimicrobial properties. The bark of a tamarind tree has an astringent action. To a glassful of infusion obtained from sage leaves, add a teaspoon of honey and 2-3 drops of vinegar. Now use this for gargling—a teaspoonful does no harm. Sage leaves have essential oils, which probably have an antifungal action too—the infusion is used as a gargle for thrush infections of the mouth and throat, and for gingivitis. Fenugreek seeds can also be used to make an infusion for gargling. They have mucilage, which has a soothing and emollient action. Its essential oils also act on the neuromuscular endings, reviving deadened taste buds—a result of a persistent sore throat.

PAIN IN THE THROAT

Any infection or inflammation of the throat will cause pain, which often causes difficulty in swallowing food or speaking.

Causes and symptoms

Sometimes a throat pain may feel like a needle pricking at a particular point. This is often because of a pus point or a small abscess waiting to burst. The remedies given earlier for sore throat will also help in alleviating the pain. Try any of them.

Remedies

- Half a cup of fresh bottle gourd juice, flavoured with honey, is soothing for pain in the throat. It has cooling properties, is a diuretic, a good source of vitamin-B complex, and a fair source of vitamin-C and magnesium. Magnesium ions relieve pain.

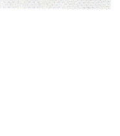

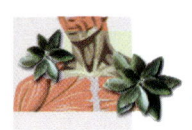

- One-third of a cup each of fresh spinach juice and carrot juice is cooling and soothing.

- One finely-cut fresh onion, flavoured with half a teaspoon of freshly roasted ground cummin seeds, with rock salt added for taste, is another remedy for pain in the throat.

- A tablespoon of the bark of the *grewia asiatica* tree, ground and boiled in two glasses of water, should be used for gargling. It is cooling as well as an astringent.

- A sherbet made from mulberry, or the fruits eaten whole, is cooling as well as rich in vitamin-C.

- Add a tablespoonful of the pounded dry bark of the mango tree to two glasses of water, make a decoction and keep aside. Add two tablespoons of this decoction to half a glass of water and gargle with it 2-3 times a day.

- Boil a handful of crushed rose petals in a glassful of water. Filter and add honey to taste, and sip it while it is still warm. It relieves soreness and pain in the throat.

HOARSENESS

Those who use their voices a great deal, or have to speak loudly most of the time, often suffer from hoarseness.

Causes and symptoms

Any infection of the throat, especially in the area of the larynx (voice box), will cause hoarseness. The home remedies for throat pain, above, as well as the following ones, can help to relieve this condition. But if there is any external swelling in the region of the throat, with no complaints suggestive of throat infection, it must be immediately investigated. Often, in the case of a benign or malignant growth in the thyroid glands (these are situated in front of the voice box), there may be some pressure being exerted on the nerve supplying the muscles of the larynx. This results in hoarseness, which must never be taken lightly or neglected.

ROSE

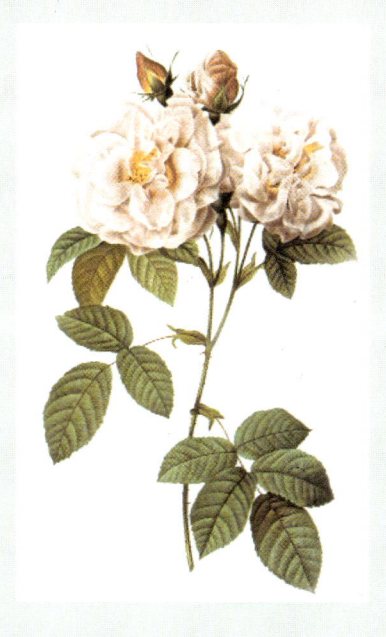

Botanical name: *Rosa centifola*

Description and uses: This particular rose, also known as cabbage rose, is known for its fragrance. It is large and rose-purple or dark pink in colour. The petals are dried and used to make rose water, oil of rose, rose syrup, rose jelly, infusions and decoctions. Its medicinal uses are many and it is used effectively in the treatment of problems relating to the head, a sore mouth, throat pain, tonsillitis, belching, diarrhoea, measles, chicken pox, skin infections, chapped lips, body odour, tanned skin and vaginal discharge.

Remedies

■ Take a white turnip. Slice it in circles horizontally and apply honey to the circles. Now sandwich them together. Hold firmly, and slice longitudinally, apply honey again, and then tie them together with a clean, washed thread—not too tight, just tightly enough to hold the pieces together. Pour some more honey over them. Leave for 12-14 hours. The turnip-honey syrup will collect at the bottom of the cup. A teaspoon of this, taken thrice a day with warm water, gives remarkable relief. Even gargling with water in which turnips have been boiled is efficacious.

■ Alternatively, a teaspoonful of onion juice, mixed with a teaspoonful of honey, is equally beneficial.

■ Gargle with an infusion of a teaspoon each of powdered cinnamon and

To make rose-petal jelly or preserve, rose petals from white roses, popularly known as summer damask rose, are plucked from the base.

■ To 400 gms sugar (about 2 1/2 cupsful), in a saucepan, add a tablespoon of lime juice. Cook on low heat till the sugar melts. Now add 100 gms rose petals and cook gently till the petals seem to dissolve. Take off the heat and let the mixture cool. Add two tablespoons of honey. Bottle and store. Have a teaspoonful 2-3 times a day. It heals chronic tonsillitis and also acts as a mild laxative. The English recipe advocates adding the honey and letting it cook along with the other ingredients. However, according to ayurveda, honey should never be cooked. It is full of enzymes that either get destroyed when cooked, or denatured into substances not conducive to good health.

■ Gather the roses, wash and wipe them, then remove the petals and add sugar to coat them well. Place in a transparent glass jar, cover tightly with a transparent cloth, and place it in the sun. The rose petals should be topped up well with sugar. Within ten days the sugar will melt and become a syrup, and the petals too will be reduced to a mash. This does not have a long shelf life, hence should be eaten within a few days.

cardamom, mixed with a glassful of water.

■ Gargle with an infusion of fennel—a teaspoon to a glass of water.

■ For relief from a chronic throat irritation, soak 2-3 dried figs and 2-3 almonds in a cup of warm water for 2-3 hours. The outer skin of the almonds softens. Remove it. Grind the almonds and figs to a fine paste. Add a teaspoon of honey to it, and drink it with a cup of warm water at bedtime. It is delicious with hot milk, but perhaps a little fattening for people who need to watch their weight!

■ Take equal quantities of liquorice and lump sugar. Grind them together and bottle the mixture. Take one-fourth to half a teaspoon at a time. Keep in the mouth, let the saliva mix with it, and swallow it slowly, a little at a time. It soothes the throat and is excellent for hoarseness of the voice. If one does not dislike the pungency of black pepper, an equal amount of it can be added. However, some find it too pungent and an irritant, instead of soothing.

TONSILLITIS/PHARYNGITIS/LARYNGITIS

These cause inflammation of specific areas of the throat. The remedies enumerated earlier will give relief, if used at the beginning of the problem. If, however, there is an overwhelming infection, these may not suffice, as they are catalysts/synergists for the inherent healing mechanisms of the body, and sometimes they are ineffective for virulent infections. Hence, expert medical attention is needed.

Remedies

■ Use pounded acacia bark to make a decoction. Add a pinch of salt and gargle—for enlarged tonsils.

■ A paste of equal quantities (one-fourth teaspoon) of mustard seeds, barley, linseed, drumstick seeds, applied locally on the tonsils like a throat paint (like the Mandel's throat paint of yesteryear), twice a day, helps reduce the inflammation and size of enlarged tonsils.

Studies have shown that mustard, drumstick seeds and oil have a distinctive antimicrobial action, whereas linseed has a mucilaginous quality, which makes it an ideal base for poultices, embrocations and linaments. Barley seeds have soothing, demulcent and mucilaginous properties. Drumstick seeds or their oil, and barley seeds, counter the sharpness of the irritation caused by the mustard paste. This preparation should be made fresh every time, and only a thin layer should be applied. It has a sharp taste and is not very palatable. Do not apply it if it causes irritation. Some people may be sensitive to mustard.

■ Dry water lettuce or tropical duckweed, and burn it to an ash. Moisten it with a drop of mustard oil, and apply a thin layer on chronic, enlarged tonsils twice a day.

■ Dried figs, boiled, softened and then mashed, and the warm paste applied to the tonsils is soothing and quite palatable too. Add honey to this, and eat the stewed figs with just a little water/ syrup—ideal for hoarseness caused by laryngitis.

■ Take 2-3 flowers of *viola odorata*, sweet violet. Wash and crush them, and boil them in a cup of milk. Strain and drink the milk while it is still hot. It relieves the pain and swelling of inflamed tonsils. The flowers are an emollient and demulcent. Even a decoction of fresh leaves—a tablespoon in a glass of warm water—relieves throat pain. These flowers can be dried in a shady place, stored, and used when needed. However, do not stretch a good thing too far as these also have a mildly laxative action in their fresh state, and a purgative one when dried!

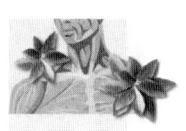

HICCUPS

A hiccup is a sharp sound which occurs due to a sudden contraction of the diaphragm, followed simultaneously by a spasm/closure of the vocal chords. This is not a disorder to worry about, but can be very uncomfortable and tiresome while it lasts. Usually it is self- limiting.

Remedies

- Take a teaspoon each of ginger juice, honey, lime juice and a pinch of pepper. Mix them together and lick a tiny bit from a spoon, off and on.

- Slowly suck on a wedge of fresh lime.

- Sip warm water slowly.

- Nibble fresh radish leaves—it stops hiccups.

CHOKING

Any obstruction in the windpipe causes choking. This usually occurs when food goes down the wrong pipe! The treatment requires a quick reaction. Standing behind the victim, grasp her or him firmly around the waist with your left hand made into a fist, the thumb extended inwards and pressed into the centre of the rib cage. With the encircling arm, the right hand now placed firmly over the left, press sharply upward and inward, making the patient cough out the offending article.

DIPHTHERIA

With improved immunisation programmes, one rarely hears of diphtheria in the developed world. But under-developed or third-world countries still battle with the disease, which usually occurs in the pre-winter or late autumn months.

Causes and symptoms

Diptheria is a serious infectious disease, caused by bacteria spread through droplet infection, i.e., from the nasal discharge or skin lesions of patients suffering from it. The points of entry are the nose, mouth, eyes, skin or genital mucous. It often lodges itself in the throat or in the upper respiratory tract, but causes generalised or localised symptoms because of a toxin it produces, which spreads through the bloodstream.

When diphtheria affects the nose or throat, it causes a blockage in the respiratory inflow. There is fever, loss of appetite, headache, and a sore throat, that rapidly turns into a breathing problem. The person begins breathing through the mouth, and gets more and more restless as time passes. Then the face puffs up and sometimes there is vomiting. There is also difficulty in swallowing. The diagnosis is confirmed by the presence of a membrane on the tonsils or throat surface, or nasal mucosa where the infection is lodged.

The best course of action is to rush to a hospital. The toxin can be neutralised with anti-toxin, along with antibiotics and other symptomatic relief measures.

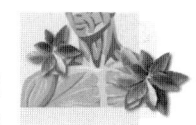

Remedies

However, if medical aid is unavailable:

- Crush 2-3 cloves of garlic and give a spoonful of the juice to the patient to drink. It should be rolled in the throat and then swallowed. If a child is unable to do this, add warm water to the juice and let him sip it slowly. Repeat this every 3-4 hours. It will disintegrate the pseudo-membrane, clear the respiratory passage, and also neutralise the circulating toxins.

The essential oils in garlic contain active sulphur compounds, allyl propyl disulphide and di-allyl disulphide. These have an efficient antimicrobial effect.

- Make a paste of 4-5 small fresh castor leaves, a handful of drumstick leaves and 3-4 cloves of garlic. Use this to make an infusion, let the patient take inhalations, and also gargle with this water.

FISH BONE IN THE THROAT

This is a common occurance, and the patient should to be rushed to hospital. However, one can try eating large chunks of dry bread, a banana or mashed potato. Often the fish bone is detached and swallowed with the food. Lemon juice with honey, sipped slowly, or gargling with a cinnamon and honey infusion, soothes the scratched throat.

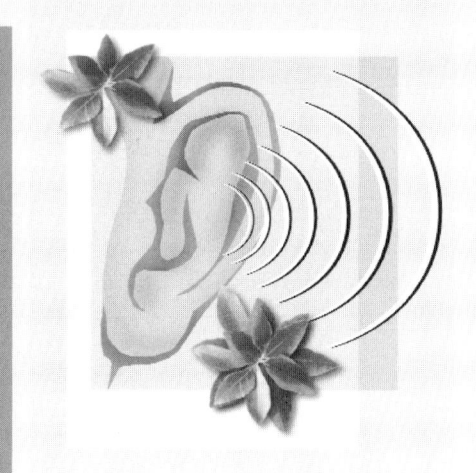

Our ears, by means of which we can hear, are intricately and delicately designed. Normally, they do not require much care, but we should ensure that they are always clean and free from infection of any kind.

■ EAR PROBLEMS

We tend to take our five senses for granted. One of these vital senses, which makes us aware of our special world, are the ears. They are our organs of hearing and balance. The hearing apparatus consists of three major parts—the external ear, the middle ear and the inner ear. Neglect of minor ear problems can lead to disastrous results. So do not neglect your ears. Here are a few common ear disorders which can be effectively handled by home remedies, thereby averting major problems.

EARACHE

An earache can be excrutiatingly painful. As the ear, nose and throat are all interconnected, the pain can also spread to these areas and cause much distress.

Causes and symptoms

Earache is usually caused by a cold getting out of hand. The ear, nose and throat are intimately connected. Any infection in one area tends to affect the other two to a lesser or greater degree. This is especially so in children. Pain can also occur if one has used a pin or matchstick to clean the ears. An erupting wisdom tooth or a toothache can also cause pain in the ear.

Remedies

- Steam inhalations often clear all the respiratory passages (ear/ nose/ throat). An infusion of eucalyptus leaves is particularly beneficial.

- A tablespoonful of mustard or sesame-seed oil, heated with a clove of garlic or a pinch of omum, then filtered and cooled to a bearable temperature, can be instilled (1-2 drops) in the ear. Tilt the head so that the oil goes into the ear, and hold the head in that position for a minute or so. Do this twice a day for 2-3 days.

- One or two drops of holy basil-leaf juice in the ear in beneficial for an earache.

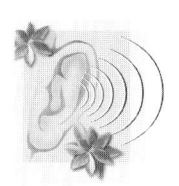

- One or two drops of garlic oil, put twice a day in the ear, is also efficacious. However, this may cause irritation in some people, so add a drop of milk to it.

- Use as a ear drop a decoction of neem leaves—1-2 drops—just warm, not hot.

- A few drops of fresh lime juice, diluted with an equal quantity of water—two drops twice a day—is also very effective.

- Ear drops can be made with the warmed fresh juice of either tender mango leaves, fresh ginger, neem leaves, or onion. Put in the ear one or two drops at a time. Do not mix these. Each remedy is individually used.

- Pound fenugreek seeds and put them in hot oil. Filter and cool it to a bearable temperature. This oil should be used as eardrops.

> DO NOT USE HAIRPINS OR TWEEZERS TO REMOVE FOREIGN BODIES IN THE EAR, AND DO NOT PUT WATER INTO THE EAR, AS SOME FOREIGN BODIES MAY SWELL UP WITH THE MOISTURE.

WAX IN THE EARS

Nature has its way of looking after our ears. There are small glands in the ear canal that produce wax. This wax entraps dust and foreign bodies, so as to leave a clear passage for the sound waves. The movements of the jaw while eating extrude the wax without our even being aware of it. Normally, cleaning the ears while bathing suffices to maintain a normal amount of wax.

Causes and symptoms

However, sometimes there is an excessive secretion, and the wax blocks the opening of the external ear canal, causing either pain or a ringing sensation in the ear, or even the sensation of not being able to hear well.

Remedy

- To remove impacted wax, put warm olive (or any other edible oil) into the ear, which will not solidify on cooling. Do this for 2-3 nights. The wax will soften and be easily removed with a ear bud.

DISCHARGE FROM THE EAR

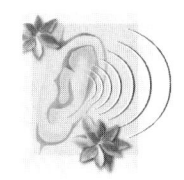

Discharge from the ear is the result of an infection and can be most troublesome. It must never be neglected.

Causes and symptoms

Any infection of the middle ear will first cause pain in the ear, and if untreated, lead to discharge from the ear. This is called otitis media. The discharge is usually pus-like but may even be bloodstained and foul-smelling. Once the discharge occurs, the pain decreases.

Remedies

As a rule, once an ear starts discharging pus nothing should be put into it. Medicine should be given orally to heal from within, e.g., antibiotics. However, in the absence of medical facilities, in case the discharge persists and becomes chronic, folk-medicine practitioners use the following remedies:

- Breast milk: A few drops of the breast milk of a healthy lactating woman can be put in an infant's infected ear. Breast milk has natural immunity-enhancing and healing properties.

- Two or three drops of warm onion juice, put in the ear 2-3 times a day, is efficacious.

- Heat a teaspoon of fenugreek seeds in a tablespoon of hot oil. Cool to a bearable temperature. Strain. A drop of this oil with a drop of fresh milk should be put in the ear to relieve a earache.

- Wash the ear with water in which neem leaves or neem bark has been boiled. This is very effective for a earache.

FOREIGN BODY IN THE EAR

Sometimes an insect gets into the ear and it is difficult to remove it. A few drops of onion juice or warm mustard oil should be instilled in the ear, and a second later the head should be tilted to the affected side. The insect and the oil will come out.

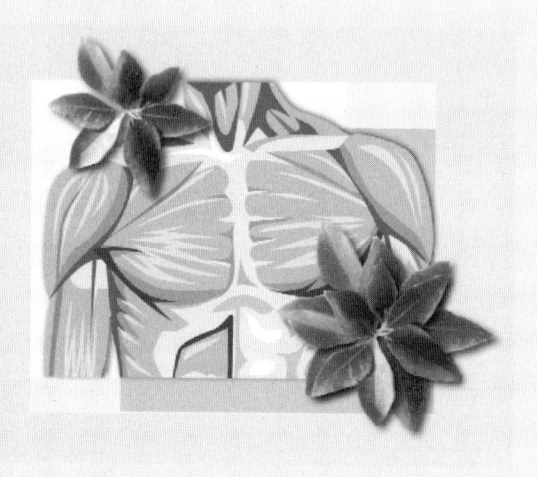

The chest encloses the heart, lung and major blood vessels. Chest pain and infection, asthma, coughs, wheezing and breathlessness are all problems which require immediate attention, as any chest problem, no matter how minor, can take a serious turn.

■ CHEST PROBLEMS

The chest is a vital part of our anatomy. It houses the heart, lungs and major blood vessels. In fact, the movement of life-giving energy is conducted from this vital site. For its protection, nature has enclosed it in the rib cage. There are various problems that can occur in this area, describing which is outside the scope of this book. However, usually there are a few symptoms which are warning signals and need to be heeded.

PAIN IN THE CHEST

Pain in the chest can be the result of chest-wall conditions, cervical spondylosis, bronchitis, pleurisy, angina, heart attack or pericarditis. Home remedies can treat mild conditions such as seasonal flu, but an anginal pain or severe chest pain should be a signal to rush to a well-equipped medical centre. There are modern drugs, which if administered within 30-40 minutes, the earlier the better, ensure that there is minimum tissue damage, and recovery is faster. Delay will cause irreparable damage.

Anginal pain

Those who suffer from angina and are under treatment could use the following complementary remedies as an adjuvant for preventing recurring attacks:

Remedies

■ Take 2-3 cloves of fresh garlic. Soak them in unboiled, fresh milk for an hour. Then eat these cloves. This should be continued in the convalescence period, after a heart attack, especially in the case of people with high blood pressure.

■ Boil 2-3 cloves of crushed garlic in a glass of milk. Drink this milk preparation once a day for a week. It is beneficial for those who have been diagnosed with actual blockage of the arteries. Under normal conditions, milk and garlic is not a good combination. It is only prescribed in special cases for short-term therapy.

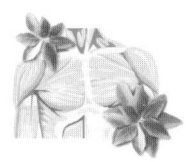

■ Two or three garlic cloves can be fried in ghee and had by patients who are not overweight.

■ Two or three cloves of garlic can be ground to a fine paste, stirred into a glass of fresh buttermilk, and drunk by the patient.

■ The diet for people diagnosed with coronary heart disease, or those recovering from a myocardial infarction must include bottle gourd or a vegetable dish made from ash gourd. Take 250 gms of bottle gourd or ash gourd. Wash well and cut into small cubes. Place in a pressure cooker with just enough water to cover. Add rock salt to taste and one-fourth to half a teaspoon of turmeric. Cook for a minute after the pressure builds up. Wait for the cooker to cool. Remove lid and season the contents with a mixture of a teaspoon each of cummin seeds and coriander seeds, roasted on a dry tawa without oil/ghee, and then ground, not very fine, but not too coarse either. Cummin seeds and coriander seeds have fibre as well as cholesterol-removing properties. Bottle gourd and ash gourd pulp have diuretic and toxin-flushing-out properties. Apparently, the debris of cholesterol and atherosclerotic plaques removed from the inner lining of the vessel wall by the action of cummin seeds, coriander and garlic, need to be removed, eliminating the possible chance of blockage in blood vessels or kidney tubules—ash gourd or bottle gourd do this.

■ Another folk remedy is to take a ripe ash gourd, and wash and cut it into small cubes. Place the cubes in an earthenware vessel and seal the lid with flour paste around the rim. Place the vessel inside an oven, and cook the ash gourd without water for 20 minutes or so. Then put the vessel aside to cool. Open the lid and take out the cooked, semi-burnt ash gourd pieces. Dry and pound them fine, and store as a powder. One teaspoon of this with a pinch of dried ginger powder should be taken daily with a glass of hot water.

■ Take a tablespoon of coriander seeds and make a decoction using a glassful of water. When half a glass remains, keep it aside to cool, and strain and filter through a muslin cloth. Prepare this decoction every day and drink it. It lowers high cholesterol levels and is also a diuretic, and so it flushes the kidneys.

- Dry roast asafoetida, cummin and omum seeds in equal measures, separately. The asafoetida releases a little water first, as it is a gum, so it is best to roast it in a non-stick pan. Then mix all three together with one-fourth of a measure of powdered rock salt to taste, i.e., 1+1+1+1/4. Store this in a dry, airtight bottle and have half a level teaspoonful daily with a glass of warm water. It is good for chest pain caused by heartburn, indigestion and flatulence—their symptoms often mimic angina.

- Herbal tea made with parsley leaves and its fruit, taken thrice a day, for those with high blood pressure or an atherosclerotic heart disease, ensures that the blood flows smoothly in the blood vessels, as parsley leaves and fruit have coumarin-like properties. Coumarin is contained in the parsley fruit, its action is anticoagulant, and hence does not allow stickiness of cellular elements in the blood—a bit like what half a Disprin does.

- *Bael*-fruit pulp or juice is a heart tonic and a cure for heart ailments. It should be taken when there is anginal pain. This too has coumarins. The juice/ pulp should not be drunk hurriedly but should be thoroughly chewed. Do not eat too much of it, as it tends to sit/settle in the stomach. This gives a feeling of heaviness and fullness, and may cause constipation and flatulence if used without a break, or if too much is taken too often.

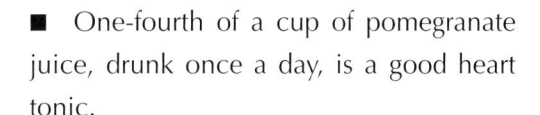

- One-fourth of a cup of pomegranate juice, drunk once a day, is a good heart tonic.

HAVING INDIAN GOOSEBERRY WHEN IT IS IN SEASON, WHOLE, OR IN CHUTNEY FORM, IS GOOD FOR THOSE WITH IRREGULAR BLOOD PRESSURE OR BLOOD PRESSURE FLUCTUATIONS. WHEN NOT IN SEASON, A DRIED GRANULE CAN BE CHEWED. IT IS AVAILABLE AS A MOUTH FRESHENER IN MODERN DEPARTMENT/GROCERY STORES. INDIAN GOOSEBERRY IS EXCEPTIONALLY HIGH IN VITAMIN-C AND BETA-CAROTENE. EVEN THE DRIED FORM HAS AS MUCH AS 2500 MG/100 GMS OF VITAMIN-C. THE FRESH FRUIT CAN BE EATEN WITH A LITTLE ROCK SALT, WHILE THE DRIED POWDER CAN BE TAKEN EITHER WITH ROCK SALT OR HONEY. IT IS AN ANTI-STRESS FOOD, WHICH KEEPS THE HEART MUSCLE HEALTHY.

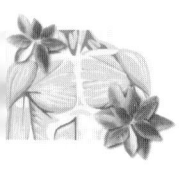

- Half a teaspoon of fresh ginger juice with half a teaspoonful of honey will relieve chest pain.

- The diet for patients suffering from heart disease should be devoid of all hot, spicy, fried food. Bitter gourd, ash gourd orange, banana, guava, apple and dry fruits are good too. Avoid hydrogenated fats. Though western medicine propagates the use of sunflower oil for cooking, ayurveda advocates only the use of ghee, made from cow's milk, as a cooking medium.

COUGH, WHEEZING, ASTHMA BREATHLESSNESS AND CHEST INFECTIONS

Cough, wheezing, asthma, breathlessness and other chest infections are all disorders of the respiratory system which require immediate remedial treatment and care.

Causes and symptoms

A cough is a sudden noisy expulsion of air from the lungs. It is a natural defence mechanism, which occurs as a reflex to help expel an irritative focus from the respiratory tract. This may be dust, chemical fumes, phlegm or a foreign body. A sneeze is like a cough, but its action is limited to getting rid of irritants from the nose.

A cough can be dry or wet. It is called dry when there is no phlegm or sputum, and can be caused by a dusty atmosphere, smelling fumes or smoke, or it can be an allergic cough, asthma, an upper respiratory-tract infection, or a common cold. In some chest infections, phlegm or pus is coughed out. This happens when the infection has progressed to the smaller divisions of the bronchial tree, or attacked lung tissue in the alveolar spaces, i.e., down at the level where gaseous exchange is taking place, e.g., in bronchitis, tuberculosis, malignancies, pneumonia, etc. Sometimes there is blood in the cough, which could be an underlying condition, a lung problem, or of cardiac origin. A cough which persists for 3-4 days, is productive, or has blood specks in the sputum, and does not get better within a day or two with herbal remedies, must be seen to by a physician. Any cough which is accompanied by chest pain, fever, difficulty in breathing, and is progressive, with diminished appetite, loss of weight and unusual fatigue, means trouble.

Wheezing is a whistling respiratory sound which occurs in asthma. In asthma, the patient has recurrent attacks of breathlessness, with wheezing and tightness in the chest, often accompanied by a dry cough. Breathing is a normal body function, which carries on all our lives without us being aware of it. When there is difficulty in breathing or laboured breathing, the effort being inappropriate to the amount of physical work being done, it is called breathlessness. In asthma, there is shortness of breath—there is intake, but breathing out is a problem. The causes of asthma are many, the underlying factor being the unusual increased response to an irritant, usually an allergen. The response is in the form of a spasm, a sustained contraction of muscles in the walls of the bronchial tree, which causes narrowing in the walls. Slowly breathing in and out becomes difficult. If it is not treated in time, the lungs overinflate, the breathing rate and heart rate both increase, and because there is no oxygen reaching the body tissue, the skin become blue, starting with the nails, lips and peripheries. The patient is agitated and frightened.

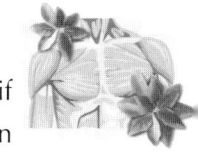

Asthma is a reversible condition, if treated in time. While an attack is in progress and sputum collects in the lungs, initially a little bit can be coughed out, but very soon that too stops, as it is thick and tenacious, blocking the respiratory passage.

With rising levels of pollution, there are more allergens in the air, and more and more people have asthma attacks. Chest infections too are common, which further precipitate attacks in susceptible people.

All cases of breathlessness, impending asthma and chest infections must be treated right at the onset.

Remedies

All the remedies for treating sore throat, tonsils, etc., will also give some relief in chest problems related to a lung infection, rather than those of cardiac origin.

For those who have repeated chest congestion/infections:

■ Take a teaspoon of ghee and fry half a teaspoon of freshly ground black pepper powder. Add two handsful of washed drumstick leaves and cook them on a low fire for 2-4 minutes. This should be eaten with hot chapatties or steaming hot rice once a day for 4-6 weeks.

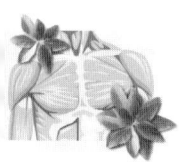

- Equal quantities of long pepper, black pepper and dried ginger should be ground together, and half a teaspoon of this taken with hot water or cow's milk. Honey can be added for taste. Have daily for 4-6 weeks.

- A fresh, tender *bael* leaf should be chewed with 2-3-peppercorns early in the morning and washed down with warm water or a cup of hot cow's milk daily for 4-6 weeks.

- To one-fourth of a level teaspoonful of powdered mustard seeds, add a teaspoon of honey and eat it once a day. Since it is very pungent it can be eaten with a chapatti or taken with warm water.

- Mix 10-12 fresh holy basil leaves, a half an inch piece of fresh ginger, 1-2 betel leaves, and grind them together. Have a teaspoon of this juice with honey 2-3 times a day for 3-4 days.

- Alternatively, boil a handful of crushed holy basil leaves in half a litre of water and reduce it to one-fourth of a litre. Take a tablespoon of this decoction with a teaspoon of honey 2-3 times a day for 3-4 days.

- Two-three holy basil leaves should be chewed with a little jaggery 3-4 times a day. (But always rinse your mouth with warm water or wash it down with it.)

- Children who are prone to chest infections can have their daily glass of milk with 8-10 leaves of holy basil boiled in it. This acts as a preventive to ward off seasonal colds when the weather changes.

- Boil a teaspoon of omum seeds in a cup of water. Add half a teaspoon of turmeric. Have one-fourth of a cup of this with a teaspoon of honey, 2-4 times a day.

- When there is a blockage of phlegm in the respiratory passage, two teaspoons of lightly roasted, crushed, coarsely powdered omum seeds in a glass of buttermilk will help clear the passage. Have this twice a day.

- Take a teaspoon each of long pepper, dried powdered ginger and cloves. Powder them together. Mix honey and make a paste. Lick this 4-5 times a day, or make an infusion with half a litre of water and drink half a cup 3-4 times a day.

- Chronic bronchitis patients should have a teaspoon of raw onion juice every morning. It liquefies blocked, dry phlegm and helps to expectorate it.

PARSLEY

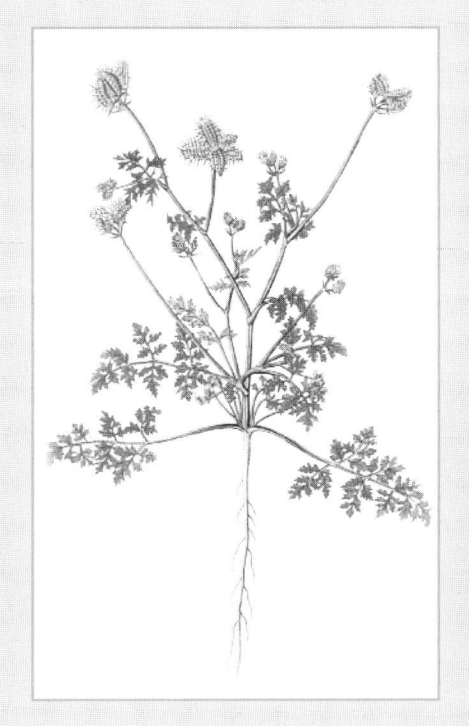

Botanical name: *Petroselinum crispum*

Description and uses: Parsley is a biennial herb, with white flowers and crinkly aromatic leaves, used for seasoning and garnishing food. Its uses, however, are many and varied, and by no means restricted to the culinary sphere. Parsley has a carminative, tonic and laxative action, and also has diuretic properties. General ailments, hypertension, chest and kidney problems, a burning sensation in passing urine, renal stones, insect bites and stings, burns, and morning sickness during pregnancy are effectively treated by this versatile herb.

■ Pound together a teaspoon each of sesame seeds and linseed. Make a decoction with a glassful of water. Boil and reduce it to half. A teaspoon of this filtrate should be taken with a teaspoon of honey twice a day. These seeds have an emollient, demulcent action. They soothe the respiratory passages and clear a cough.

■ Soak for a few hours 6-7 almonds in water. Discard the skin, grind and have almonds with half a cup of orange juice or a tablespoon of lemon juice every night.

■ Herbal tea made with fennel is also soothing for a persistent cough with difficult expectoration. It breaks up the thick tenacious mucus.

■ Dried Indian gooseberry powder (half teaspoon) mixed with a teaspoon of honey should be taken every morning with warm water. If the fresh fruit is available, grind a small segment, say a one-fourth-inch piece, and have it with a teaspoon of honey twice a day. Honey and Indian gooseberry are specially beneficial for all chest infections. Indian gooseberry is rich in vitamin-C, and honey liquefies the dried secretions so that they can be coughed out. It also soothes the throat.

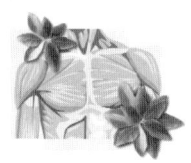

■ Add a teaspoon of linseed decoction to a glass of water. Boil and reduce it to one-fourth of a glass, strain. A tablespoon of this should be taken with a tablespoon of milk once a day. It relieves congestion and also prevents recurrence of asthma attacks. Take for 3-4 days.

■ If you have bitter gourd growing in your garden, take the root of the plant—an inch of it will do. Wash well and grind it to a fine paste with 8-10 holy basil leaves. Strain and add a teaspoon of honey. Have every night for 10-15 days.

■ Take half a teaspoon of grated ginger and 2-3 crushed cloves of garlic. Add a cupful of milk and boil. Do not use fresh, unboiled milk as it will curdle. Use milk which has been boiled once. Strain and have twice a day. It works best in aborting an attack in the early stages. Some may, however, find this too spicy and an irritant for the stomach.

■ An infusion of a teaspoon of grated ginger and a teaspoon of pounded fenugreek seeds in a glass of hot water should be filtered and drunk as tea twice a day. This is helpful for asthma.

■ Eating shredded raw cooked cabbage is good for asthma too. Having a tablespoon of raw cabbage juice, or just eating cabbage leaves when an attack is likely to occur, either helps abort it or reduces its intensity.

■ For chronic asthmatics: Take large dried grapes (the seedless variety), wash and keep them aside. Put one in your mouth, chew and swallow it. Chew slowly so that you have one of these in your mouth throughout your waking hours. This can be irritating, so have them 4-5 times a day. One will last for 20-25 minutes if chewed slowly. It acts as a lubricant and demulcent for the throat and soothes a coughing bout.

■ Thoroughly wash 4-5 figs and soak in warm water overnight. Drink the water first thing in the morning and eat the figs. Continue for 4-6 weeks. These are very

HOLY BASIL

Botanical name: *Ocimum santum*

Description and uses: Holy basil is a low, bushy plant with ovate leaves and flowers in whorls towards the top of the branches. The leaves are fragrant and aromatic and are valuable as remedies for a variety of ailments. The leaves of the holy basil lead the home-herbal list as a febrifuge. Their anti-inflammatory and analgesic properties are well researched and documented. They relieve pain, clear respiratory passages of congestion, and are excellent as a remedy for change of season fevers, cholera, piles, kidney problems, fungal infections, pimples, nausea and vomiting, hypertension, sore throats, earache, coughs, asthma, breathlessness, indigestion, dyspepsia and biliousness.

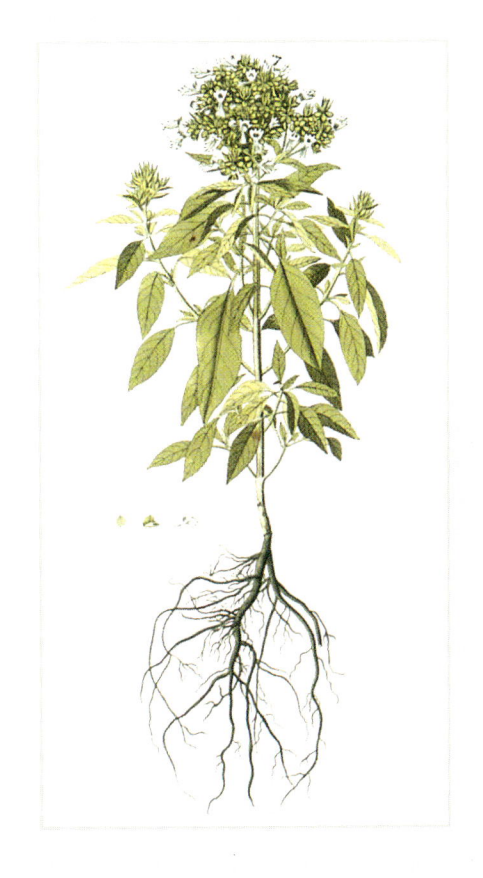

rich in trace elements like zinc and copper. Copper is also supposed to benefit those who have a constitutional tendency to asthma, hence the practice of storing drinking water in copper vessels.

■ A glass of hot milk with a teaspoon each of turmeric and honey is exceptionally soothing and relieves congestion and cough. This acts best on an empty stomach.

Inhalation

Steam or eucalyptus-leaf-infusion inhalations are extremely beneficial for any chest/ lung condition.

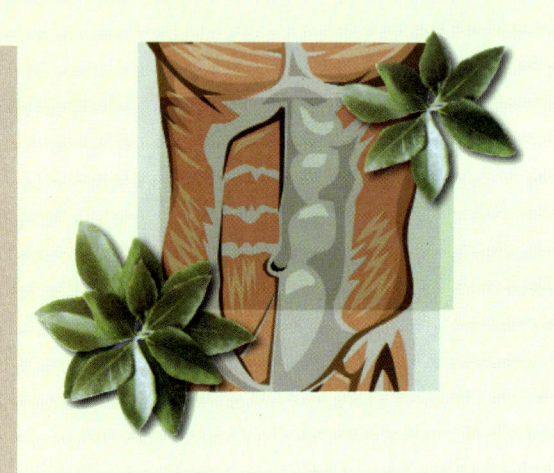

All the organs involved in the digestive process are enclosed in the abdomen. They are the foodpipe, the stomach, the small and large intestines, the liver, the gall bladder and the pancreas. All infections or ailments of any of these organs totally disrupt the entire system, and hence should be treated right at the onset.

ABDOMINAL DISORDERS

The abdomen houses all the organs that are responsible for the digestive processes, from digestion to processing and assimilation. The organs involved are the foodpipe or oesophagus, the stomach, the intestines—small and large—the liver and gallbladder, and the pancreas. The beginning of this gartronomic journey actually starts from the mouth, where the teeth masticate the food with rolling movements of the tongue, and the secretions of the salivary glands in the mouth covert it all into a smooth bolus, which goes into the foodpipe. Most of the complaints related to the abdomen are caused by dietary indiscretions or by infections. Some, of course, are constitutional in nature, with inborn/genetic tendencies. Here we will only deal with palliatives which can provide symptomatic relief. Dietary indiscretions, and the complaints emanating from them, will benefit, but constitutional or metabolic disorders are beyond the scope of this book. However, the remedies will still complement orthodox medical treatment.

HYPERACIDITY AND HEARTBURN

In today's fast-paced and stressful world, where people have the wrong kind of food and drink, often 'on the run', hyperacidity and heartburn are common problems which are rampant.

Causes and symptoms

In hyperacidity or heartburn, a person feels a burning pain in the gullet or chest—a feeling of regurgitation of the acidic contents of the stomach. Sometimes there is associated belching, which seems to relieve the immediate discomfort. The causes of this are many, but the usual culprits are overeating, eating too much spicy, rich and oily food, excessive alcohol consumption, or smoking too much. Sometimes this complaint is caused by stooping or lying down immediately after a meal, and is worse when lying on the right

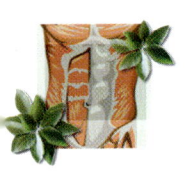

HONEY

Description and uses: Honey is a sweet, sticky yellowish fluid made by bees from nectar collected by them from flowers. It is used in many sweets and desserts and is also a valuable herbal remedy. Honey is used to treat multifarious ailments such as fever, problems related to the head, eyes and nose, anaemia, nausea and vomiting, dizziness and fainting, hypertension, a sore mouth, hoarseness, tonsillitis, pharyngitis, hippups, fish bones stuck in the throat, chest pains, coughs, wheezing, asthma, breathlessness, chest infections, hyperacidity and heartburn, flatulence, constipation, diarrhoea, cholera, jaundice, piles, intestinal worms, renal stones, diabetes, arthritis, chilblains, boils, fungal infections, freckles, spots, acne, allergic rashes, warts, wounds, burns, ant bites, bee and wasp stings, dog bites, stress-related disorders, sexual debility, gynaecological problems, and irregular or excessive menstruation.

side. The latter condition is due to a reflux of stomach contents into the oesophagus or foodpipe, because the sphincter or valve at the lower end of the foodpipe and entrance to the stomach is weak. It is supposed to be a one-way valve, but weakness of the circular muscles at the lower end of the oesophagus causes it to remain open, so the stomach contents regurgitate upwards into the chest and mouth. Heartburn may not merely be a burning, uncomfortable sensation, but may cause chest pain mimicking a heart attack. The symptoms need investigation if they are not apparently due to a dietary indiscretion, as they may be the first sign of an ulcer in this area.

Remedies

■ Boil half a teaspoon of dried Indian gooseberry with half a teaspoon of dried *terminalia chebula* in a cupful of water. Filter and cool it. Tempered with honey and sipped, it helps relieve heartburn.

■ Soak 2-3 fresh, washed *bael* leaves in a cupful of water. Pour into a copper container. Leave overnight and drink it the next morning. Continue this for 4-6 weeks. If there is no copper vessel available, it can be kept in a normal glass container.

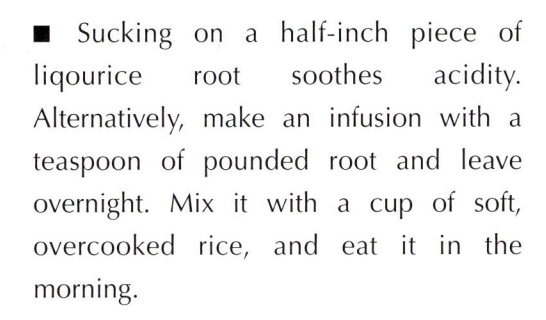

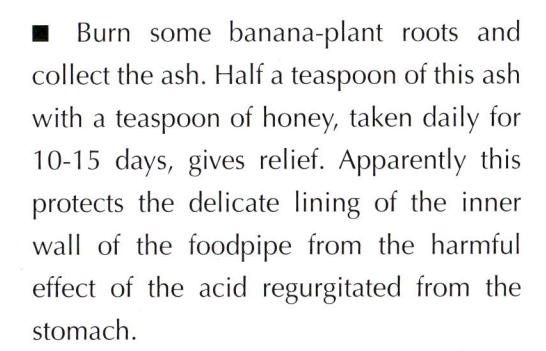

- Sucking on a half-inch piece of liquorice root soothes acidity. Alternatively, make an infusion with a teaspoon of pounded root and leave overnight. Mix it with a cup of soft, overcooked rice, and eat it in the morning.

- Burn some banana-plant roots and collect the ash. Half a teaspoon of this ash with a teaspoon of honey, taken daily for 10-15 days, gives relief. Apparently this protects the delicate lining of the inner wall of the foodpipe from the harmful effect of the acid regurgitated from the stomach.

- Eating a ripe, mashed banana with a cup of milk in the morning has a soothing effect on heartburn and stomach ulcers.

- Having a teaspoonful of psyllium husk fibre with 2-3 tablespoons of milk immediately after a meal prevents this reflux.

- If there is heartburn at other times, not just after meals, drink half a cup of fresh, sweet orange juice to which a pinch of rock salt is added. This will bring immediate relief.

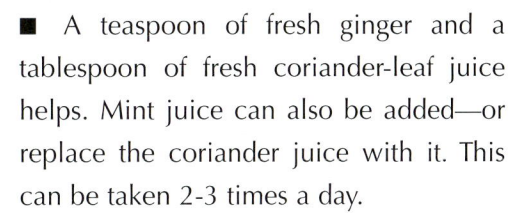

- A teaspoon of fresh ginger and a tablespoon of fresh coriander-leaf juice helps. Mint juice can also be added—or replace the coriander juice with it. This can be taken 2-3 times a day.

- A teaspoon of fresh ginger juice with a teaspoon of freshly roasted, coarsely ground cummin seeds, and a pinch of rock salt, all added to a glass of buttermilk, is a particularly soothing drink for heartburn.

- Mix a teaspoonful of fresh ginger juice with a similar amount of honey. Lick it from a spoon now and then, 2-3 times a day.

- Lightly roast omum seeds and add an

Note: *Repeated attacks of heartburn should be investigated. A heartburn associated with pain in the neck and left shoulder, and shortness of breath, could actually be angina or a heart attack. It may also be a stomach ulcer, especially if there is associated vomiting with blood.*

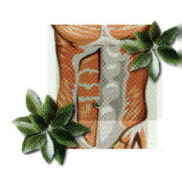

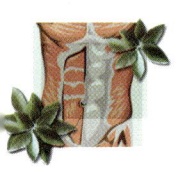

equal quantity of rock salt. Grind finely to a powder and bottle. One-fourth to half a teaspoon of this mixture, taken with hot water 2-3 times a day, relieves acidity. A pinchful can also be taken without water. It clears the taste in the mouth and relieves heartburn.

■ Take a spoonful each of dry coriander and cummin seeds. Pound them coarsely, add half a litre of water and leave overnight. In the morning, mash the seeds in the water and then filter. Add jaggery or sugar to taste, and have 2-3 tablespoons twice a day for 4-5 days.

INDIGESTION / DYSPEPSIA / BILIOUSNESS

Indigestion, dyspepsia or biliousness are usually brought on by overeating, and cause acute discomfort in the throat, chest and abdomen.

Causes and symptoms

There is a feeling of heaviness in the abdomen; that the undigested food is still in the stomach. This is accompanied by loss of appetite, nausea, regurgitation of sour fluids from the stomach, flatulence, and excessive salivation. Irregular eating hours, eating too much or too fast after having missed a meal, or just eating for want of anything better to do—the food being rich, spicy, oily, or what is known as 'junk food'—cause these problems.

Remedies

■ Eat regular well-spaced meals. Eat only when you are hungry, and eat a little less than what you feel like having.

■ Limit your fluid intake when you have solid food. Do not eat fast, but chew your food thoroughly in a relaxed manner. You don't have a train to catch, and neither is food going out of fashion!

■ Eat plenty of greens and wholegrain carbohydrates, restrict the intake of refined carbohydrates like maida and white flour, and also spices and fried food. Eat the right combination of foods.

■ If milk causes indigestion, you may have lactose intolerance. Avoid milk and milk products. If you do not have lactose intolerance or milk allergy, and it is only an infrequent problem, have a tablespoon of lime juice with a little water.

■ Sipping hot water relieves the feeling of fullness and indigestion.

■ Grind the dried rind / peel of pomegranate fine and store it in a dry bottle. Have half a teaspoonful thrice a day or after meals.

■ Make a decoction of half a teaspoon each of cloves and black pepper seeds, a tablespoon of cummin seeds, one-fourth of a teaspoon of turmeric, and half a teaspoon of rock salt, coarsely pounded, in a litre of water. Boil it down to half a litre, filter and keep aside to cool. Take two tablespoons of this mixture 3-4 times a day. It can be kept in a refrigerator for 2-3 days, but do not have it cold—have it at room temperature.

■ A herbal tea made with a teaspoon of pounded fenugreek seeds in a cup of water allays biliousness.

■ Thin buttermilk seasoned with dry, roasted, coarsely crushed cummin seeds and grated fresh ginger, with salt and black pepper to taste, is also extremely soothing for a dyspeptic, rumbling stomach.

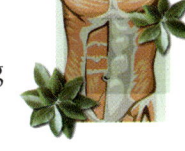

■ Mint or fennel leaves can be used to make herbal teas or infusions. These are very 'cooling' for the stomach.

■ Do not eat fruits just before or after a meal.

■ Half a cup of fresh pineapple or pomegranate juice is a good digestive.

■ Take a tablespoon of holy basil juice, a teaspoon of dried ginger powder, and twice the amount of jaggery. Mix the three ingredients well and take half a teaspoon twice a day with warm water. This helps digestion and regulates the appetite.

For storing: *Coarsely pound a measure each of coriander seeds and cummin seeds, one-fourth measure of cloves, one-fourth measure of black pepper, and store. When needed, half a teaspoon of this mixture, boiled in half a cup of water with a pinch of turmeric and salt, is a herbal tea which is easy to prepare.*

The following remedies are effective if indigestion is episodic—a once-in-a-while affair after eating a particular food.

- If you have eaten too much rice at a meal and are feeling full, sip a glass of hot water slowly.

- For indigestion caused by eating cucumber (some people cannot digest cucumber and keep regurgitating its taste), do not peel it. Slice the end and rub it on the cut surface till white froth comes out. This removes the bitterness. Do not peel—use as a salad without peeling it. The peel has ingredients which counteracts this particular effect. Munching a few grains of roasted wheat or coarsely pounded wheat porridge helps overcome this complaint.

- If one has eaten too many mangoes, as often happens during the mango season, sip half cup of cow's milk. It is very efficacious.

- Indigestion caused by eating jackfruit is relieved by eating a banana.

- Have grewia (fruit) or ripe bael, followed by a little neem juice, or chew on fresh neem leaves after eating the fruit. It is effective in relieving indigestion.

- Indigestion caused by eating palm fruit or coconut is relieved by having a little cooked rice.

- Indigestion caused by overeating sweets, fried foods, etc., is alleviated by chewing on long pepper seeds.

- *Khichri,* a dish made with rice and pulses, is often eaten as a light meal. *Khichri* made with split moong dal is light and easy to digest, whereas with other dals it is heavy. The feeling of heaviness after eating it is relieved by having a pinch of rock salt.

- One-fourth to half a cup of fresh pomegranate juice, or a pinch of the dried powdered rind of the fruit, is also a good digestive.

- Take equal quantities of powdered dried ginger, black pepper, long pepper and rock salt. Mix well and store. A pinch of this after a heavy meal helps digestion.

- If indigestion causes a stomach ache, take half a teaspoon of the mixture of equal quantities of fresh holy basil and ginger juice every 3-4 hours. It is very effective and can be taken with warm water too.

- Take the pulp of a ripe bael fruit—this will be about three-fourth of a cup to one cup. Add half a cup of tamarind pulp and half a cup of yoghurt. Mix well and churn in a liquidiser. Now mix enough water to make it palatable and not sour. A little jaggery and rock salt can be added for taste. Strain this sherbet and have thrice a day for a day. This will clear the bowels in a gentle fashion, and the heavy bloated feeling in the abdomen will disappear. Ripe *bael* pulp has a laxative action. The sourness of tamarind stimulates the digestive juices, and yoghurt replenishes the lactobacillus in the intestines, which are sluggish or have been washed away following the laxative action.

MINT

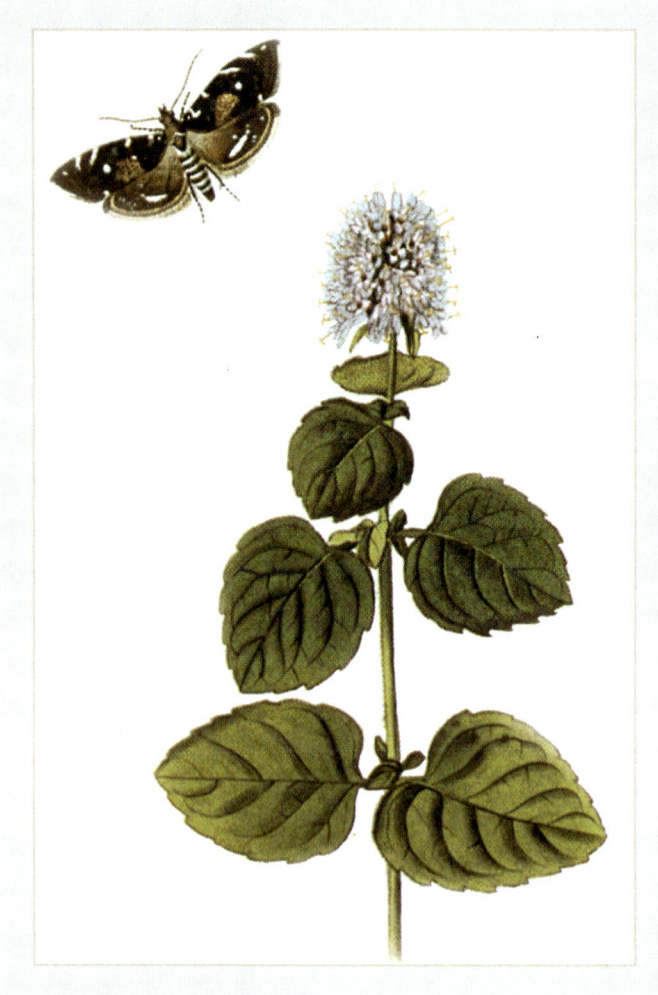

Botanical name: *Mentha spicata*

Description and uses: Mint shrubs are about 2-feet high, bearing short-stalked, lance-shaped, wrinkled, bright green leaves, with fine-toothed edges and prominent ribs beneath. The leaves are not only used for culinary purposes, but have a stimulant, carminative and antispasmodic action. Mint relieves hiccups, flatulence and indigestion. It is an excellent remedy for fevers, inflammation, problems related to the head, dizziness and fainting, nose problems, hyperacidity and heartburn, dyspepsia, irritable bowel syndrome, diarrhoea, jaundice, muscle strains and sprains, fungal infections of the skin, allergic rashes and stress-related disorders. It allays nausea, vomiting and colic, and soothes haemorrhoids. Mint also has febrifugal and diuretic properties, and is an essential ingredient in herbal tooth powder.

BELCHING / GAS IN ABDOMEN / FLATULENCE

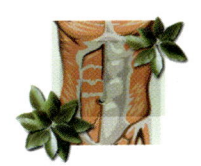

Belching, gas in the abdomen and flatulence are embarrassing problems suffered by many people. They are linked to hyperacidity and heartburn.

Causes and symptoms

Eating or drinking too fast, gulping or guzzling aerated soft drinks, nervous swallowing of air, or smoking, can result in a noisy return of air from the stomach to the mouth. This is called belching. Gas in the abdomen, known as wind, occurs due to fermentation of food in the intestines, giving a bloated feeling and the embarrassing passage of wind from the anus called flatulence. When there is ingestion of the wrong kinds of food and indigestion, the gas expelled is foul smelling.

Remedies

■ The age-old remedy of taking Eno's Fruit Salt for gas in the abdomen is still applicable. If you do not have it at home, make your own. Too much of it can cause rebound acidity—so do not make it a habit.

Mix together half a teaspoon of cooking soda or baking powder, a tablespoon of fresh lime juice, and a teaspoon of fresh ginger juice, in a glass of water and drink it. You can mix half a teaspoon of baking soda and dried ginger powder and have it with hot water before your meal, if you habitually have flatulence. (This has a high amount of sodium ions, hence is not good for those with hypertension.)

■ Soak two cloves of crushed garlic in a glass of hot water for 2-3 minutes. Add a spoonful of ginger juice and drink it while it is still warm. Leave the dregs of crushed garlic in the glass.

■ A teaspoon of turmeric in a glass of hot water, with a pinch of rock salt, drunk while still hot, gives immediate relief.

■ A teaspoon of crushed omum seeds with a few drops of lime juice, washed down with warm water, gives relief.

■ Grind together and store 100 gms omum, 100 gms dry ginger and 25 gm rock salt. This can be taken when needed—a level teaspoon of the mixture with warm water. It can be made into a soothing drink by adding a tablespoon of fresh lime juice.

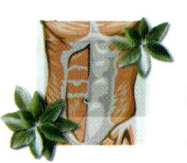

- Take 100 gms omum and 100 gms dried ginger. Soak in 250 ml of fresh lime juice. Let it dry. Powder fine. Add 25 gms of rock salt, mix and take a pinch when needed, on the tongue with a little water.

- Make herbal tea with a teaspoon of fenugreek seeds, 4-6 crushed cloves and a glass of water. Boil to make a tea. Strain. The softened cloves can also be eaten with the tea.

- Take 2-3 bay leaves and the peel of half an orange. Allow them to simmer in a glass of boiling water for 4-5 minutes. Strain/ filter and drink.

- Chewing a cardamom pod after a meal, or making tea with the seeds of 3-4 crushed pods, a pinch of dried ground ginger, and a small pinch of grated nutmeg, will settle a flatulent, rumbling stomach. Do not make having nutmeg a habit. It is addictive and constipating and has cummulative toxic effects.

- An infusion of fennel or chewing a teaspoon of roasted fennel is a good digestive.

- To make mint tea, add a teaspoon of dried herbs, or a tablespoon of fresh crushed herb to a cup of boiling water. Simmer for a few minutes. Filter and drink it at a temperature you like. This relieves flatulence and pain.

- Chewing on a small crushed betel leaf with a few drops of honey relieves gas.

- The use of asafoetida while cooking gas-producing vegetables or pulses has a purpose. Gas-producing vegetables are onion, cabbage, broccoli, turnips and beans, and fruits like melons and raw apples. Soak pulses in water 2-3 hours before cooking. This eliminates gas-producing toxins and also decreases overall cooking time.

- To tamarind water, i.e., the soft extract of tamarind boiled with a glass of water, add sugar to taste and a teaspoonful of

> THE PRACTICE OF HAVING BETEL LEAF (*PAAN*) WITH FENNEL, PEPPERMINT, CLOVE, CARDAMOM, ROSE JELLY, CATECHU AND QUICKLIME AID DIGESTION. HAVING A *PAAN AFTER* A MAJOR MEAL HELPS DIGESTION, BUT HAVING ONE EVERY HALF AN HOUR IS COUNTERPRODUCTIVE AND MAY LEAD TO ORAL CANCER.

mildly roasted crushed cummin seeds. This will settle flatulence.

- For persistent indigestion and flatulence drink a cup of goat's milk. However, goat's milk is not easily available in towns and cities, with pasteurised dairy milk being the order of the day, so you can substitute goat's milk with cow's milk.

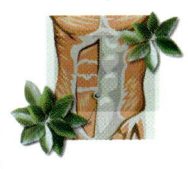

COLIC/CRAMPS IN THE ABDOMEN

Colic is an acute paroxysmal pain and a feeling of discomfort in the abdomen which causes great distress.

Causes and symptoms

Colic is caused by an accumulation of gas in the large intestine, a result of poor digestion, fermentation, etc. It can also occur due to kidney or gallbladder stones. Colic caused by indigestion will respond to herbal home remedies, but gallbladder or kidney stones will need more specific cures.

Remedies

- Have a teaspoon of fresh ginger juice with a teaspoon of fresh lime juice and a pinch of rock salt and a little sugar. It can also be taken with a little warm water.

- A tablespoon of crushed, fresh, tamarind leaves ground to a paste with one-fourth teaspoon of rock salt, mixed in half a cup of water, relieves colic.

- A teaspoon of omum seeds, crushed or pounded coarsely, with a pinch of rock salt added, relieves colic or any indigestion-related pain. To this can be added half a cup of ripe *bael*-fruit pulp and jaggery to taste, in case there is constipation.

- A tablespoon of fresh radish juice mixed with equal amounts of fresh lime juice, diluted with a little water, is also another effective remedy for colic. The practice of eating radish flavoured with lime juice as a salad is probably because of its digestive properties.

Note: *For acute pain in the abdomen, oral intake of solid food should be stopped. Only fluids should be given in small, spaced amounts till the cause is identified. Do not give an enema. The remedies cited above are all liquid. If there is no relief, see a doctor immediately.*

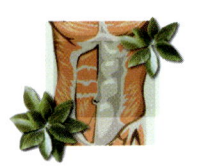

CONSTIPATION

In constipation there are infrequent, irregular or difficult bowel movements, which result in the bowel not being emptied of the waste products of digestion.

Causes and symptoms

Constipation is associated with a general feeling of malaise, loss of appetite, headache, depression, ulcers in the mouth, a coated tongue, bad breath, pimples, acne, acidity, heartburn and disturbed sleep. According to ayurveda; digestive waste products not being eliminated causes an accumulation of toxins in the system, which results in systemic disorders like arthritis, high blood pressure, etc.

Constipation is often caused by not heeding the call of nature in time. A sedentary lifestyle, irregular eating habits, an incorrect diet, a disturbed and worried mind, drinking too much tea or coffee, smoking, the excessive intake of alcoholic beverages, all add up to a sluggish digestion, stasis and overloading of the colon, ineffectual evacuation, and finally, chronic constipation.

Remedies

■ Drink a glass of warm water early in the morning, walk around for a while, and then visit the toilet. The water sets up peristalsis, and walking around braces up the system. Do not be in a rush to go to work. Instead wake up early, so that there is enough time for everything.

■ Eat a lot of raw salads and green vegetables. Drink plenty of water, but not immediately before or after a meal.

■ Drink a glassful of warm water with a spoonful of honey every night before going to sleep. (This may not be a good idea for those with a weak bladder.)

■ Have a glass of warm water with fresh lime in the morning.

■ Eat half a cupful of the pulp of a ripe *bael* fruit and a teaspoon of jaggery every day in the evening before dinner. For chronic constipation have this regularly for 4-6 weeks.

■ The ripe pulp of *bael* fruit can also be made into a pleasant sherbet. To a tablespoon of ripe *bael* pulp, add a tablespoon of tamarind water and half a teaspoon of jaggery, and drink this once

BAEL

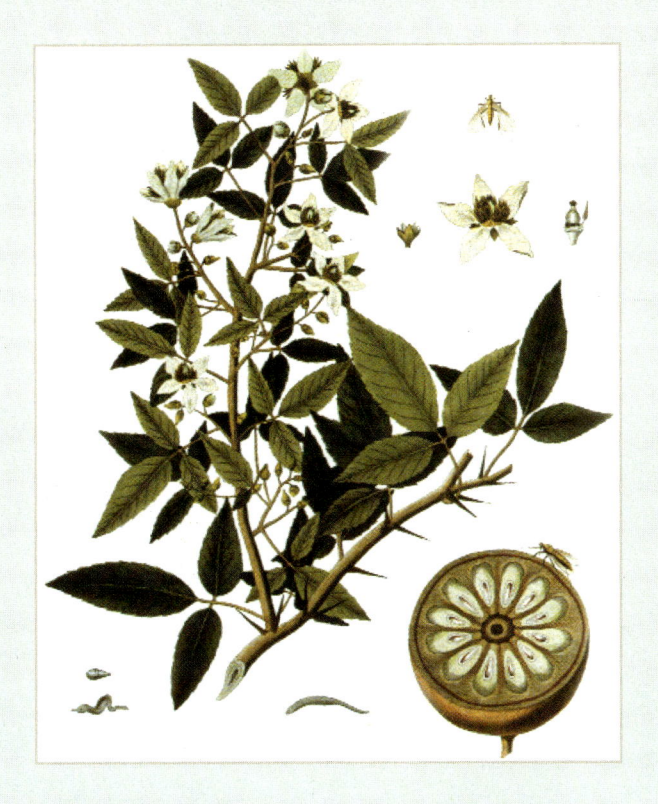

Botanical name: *Aegle marmelos*

Description and uses: The bael fruit is globular in shape, dull greenish-brown in colour, and its external surface is hard and nearly smooth. It has a thick rind, which adheres to a light red pulp inside. The pulp contains several woolly seeds, has a faintly aromatic odour and a sweet, mucilaginous taste. Fresh or dried bael pulp is considered a panacea for digestive disorders, and is also used to treat various other ailments such as fever, nausea and vomiting, hypertension, eye problems, chest pains, hyperacidity and heartburn, dyspepsia, flatulence, constipation, jaundice and excessive menstruation.

CARDAMOM

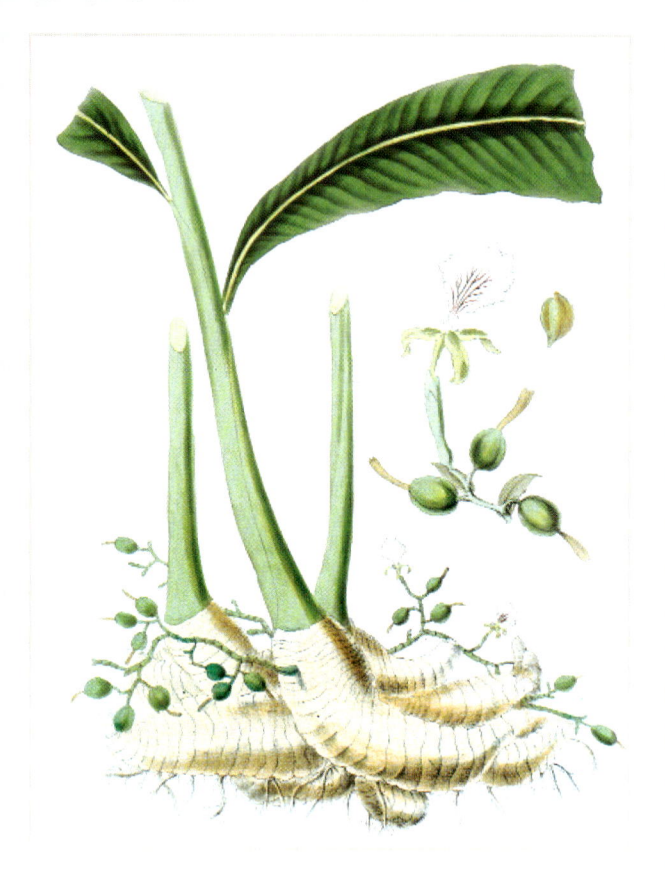

Botanical name:
Elettaria cardamomum

Description and uses: Cardamom is known in its own country, India, as *elaichi*. The plant has a large, fleshy rhizome, and the alternate, lanceolate leaves are large, smooth and dark green above, and pale, glaucous green and silky beneath. The fruits are less than an inch long and have cells inside which contain small dark, reddish-brown seeds. These fruits are dried and only the aromatic seeds are used to flavour food and for medicinal purposes. They are usually powdered just prior to use as they lose their aroma if stored as powder. Cardamom is a carminative and stimulant and is usually used as an adjuvant. As a remedy it is used to treat indigestion, flatulence, fever, nausea, vomiting, hypertension, eye disorders, chest pains, hyperacidity and heartburn, dyspepsia, constipation, amoebiasis, diarrhoea, excessive menstruation and jaundice.

or twice a day for 2-3 days. This clears chronic constipation within 2-3 days.

■ For indigestion with constipation and a stomach ache, have the diluted, ripe pulp of the *bael* fruit (half a cup of pulp with half a cup of water). Add two ground black peppercorns, a pinch of asafoetida, and half a teaspoon of pounded omum seeds. Stir well, add a teaspoon of cream, and drink this twice a day. It will clear an obstinate colon and also relieve the discomfort of indigestion.

Note: *The use of a purgative leads to potassium depletion. Bael fruit is rich in potassium (600 mg/100 grams), so it maintains the electrolyte balance. Potassium is to soft tissues what calcium is to bones!*

■ Cummin and curry-leaf chutney with rice: Take a handful of dry curry leaves. Add a teaspoon each of cummin seeds, black pepper and dried ginger powder and mix them well. Sprinkle it on half to three-fourth of a cupful of hot ghee. Add salt to taste. Mix and pour on well-cooked, soft, boiled rice. This is extremely tasty and nourishing and clears the bowels.

■ Slice a cupful of fresh onion shoots and fry them in a tablespoon of ghee. Eat them with your food. This will prevent fermentation and putrefaction in the intestines and eliminate waste matter.

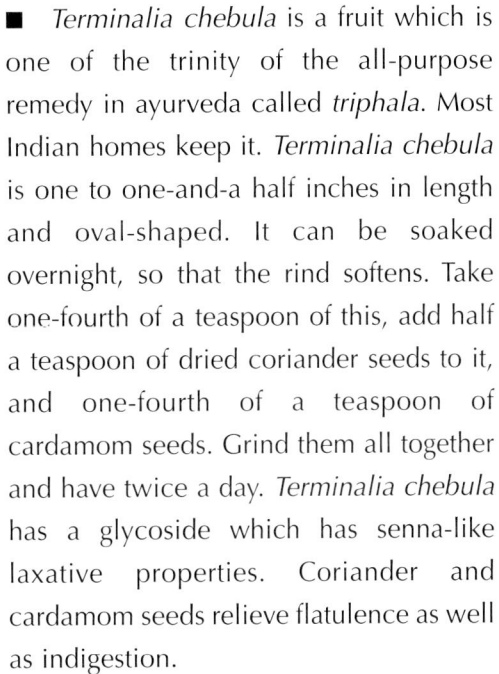

■ *Terminalia chebula* is a fruit which is one of the trinity of the all-purpose remedy in ayurveda called *triphala*. Most Indian homes keep it. *Terminalia chebula* is one to one-and-a half inches in length and oval-shaped. It can be soaked overnight, so that the rind softens. Take one-fourth of a teaspoon of this, add half a teaspoon of dried coriander seeds to it, and one-fourth of a teaspoon of cardamom seeds. Grind them all together and have twice a day. *Terminalia chebula* has a glycoside which has senna-like laxative properties. Coriander and cardamom seeds relieve flatulence as well as indigestion.

■ The softened pulp of one *terminalia chebula* can be fried in a little ghee. Add half a teaspoon of rock salt to it. Dry grind it to a powder and keep aside. A pinch of this, taken at bedtime with a cup of hot water, will clear the bowels in the morning.

■ Take a teaspoon of powdered liquorice root. Add a teaspoon of jaggery, and drink it with a cup of warm water.

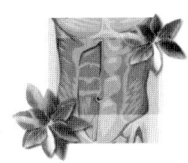

■ Roast and coarsely pound fennel and bottle them. Take half a teaspoon after meals. This acts as a good digestive.

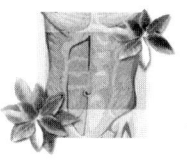

- A teaspoonful of slightly roasted fennel, taken at bedtime with a glass of warm water, acts as a mild laxative.

- Fresh or dried Indian gooseberry can be taken with a little honey (if fresh take one-fourth of a small fruit). Grind it to a paste, add honey or sugar. If dry, soak 1-2 small pieces overnight. Mash and eat the filtrate with a spoonful of honey. Drink a glass of warm water with it.

- Spinach, beetroot or fenugreek leaves, cooked as vegetables with green onion stalks, are very good for clearing the bowels. If you eat beetroot or its leaves, your urine may become reddish in colour.

- Apples, ripe bananas, papayas, oranges, ripe mangoes, grapes, pears are fruits which have a decided laxative action. Eating them regularly ensures smooth bowel action.

- Dried figs and almonds are also effective for treating chronic constipation. Soak 2-3 dried figs and 2-3 almonds for a couple of hours. Stone the figs, remove the skin of the almonds, mash them together, and have them with honey twice a day.

- Some of us are familiar with the old boarding-school remedy for constipation—a tablespoon of castor oil last thing on Saturday night ensures regular motions throughout the week. If it is too unpalatable, have it with half a cup of orange juice or milk.

- Another gentle laxative is china grass. This is a dried seaweed, which when cut into bits and cooked in milk becomes a gelatinous substance. It is used to make a milk custard-like pudding. While cooking, add sugar and flavouring to taste, and set. It makes a good vegetarian pudding and sets at room temperature. It can also be used to thicken soups or jellies. The laxative action is very gentle—ideal for children.

Note: *Diabetics should not have fruits which are sweet, including dried figs. All white foods cause constipation—white refined flour (maida), white rice, white bread, cakes, pastries, sugar, cheese and milk products.*

LIQUORICE

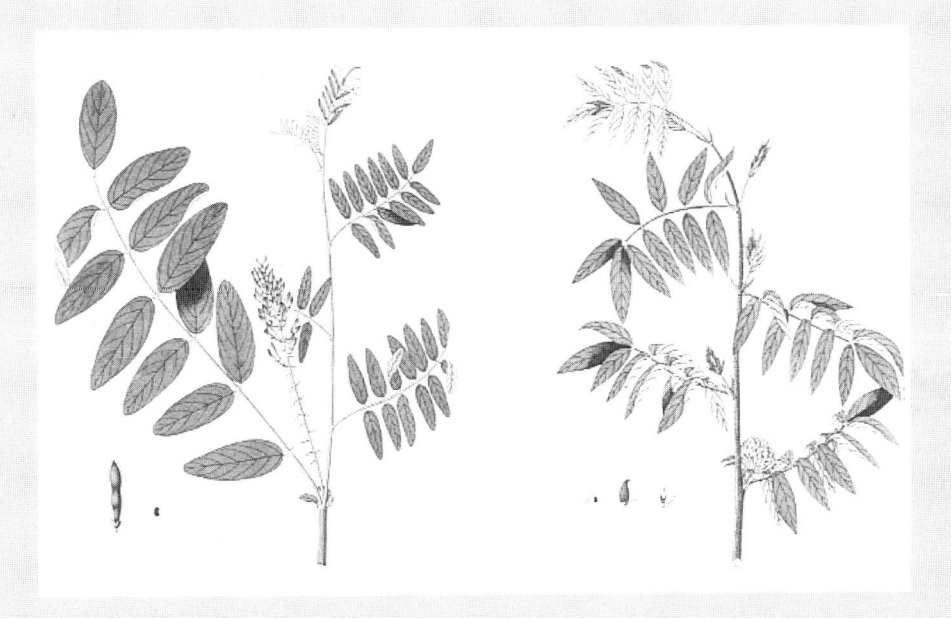

Botanical name:
Glycyrrhiza glabra

Description and uses: The uses of the liquorice plant was first introduced to Europe by the ancient Greeks, who learnt it from the Scythians. Liquorice is the black root extract of the leguminous plant *glycyrrhiza glabra*. It is used as a sweet and also in medicines. Liquorice is a demulcent and an emollient, and a well-known remedy for coughs and chest complaints, notably bronchitis. It is an ingredient used in cough medicines, sedatives and expectorants, on account of its valuable soothing properties.

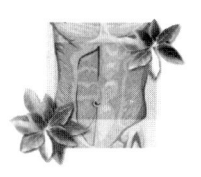

IRRITABLE BOWEL SYNDROME

Irritable bowel syndrome means just that—an irritable, stressed-out bowel. It is usually the result of mental tension causing physical stress, and is also known as a spastic colon.

Causes and symptoms

In irritable bowel syndrome one has cramp-like abdominal pains, a bloated abdomen, constipated stools alternating with diarrhoea, and passage of gas. The exact cause is not known but various theories abound. The most prevalent one is that stress not only precipitates this condition, but contributes to its severity. Women have a tendency to fall victim to it more easily than men, because they have a tendency to internalise problems.

Remedies

■ An infusion made of a handful of mint leaves (taken warm) relieves intestinal spasms and gas. Take half a cup of this infusion every few hours, 3-4 times.

■ Crushed psyllium-seed husk is a natural laxative. Again, this is something most Indian housewives buy with their monthly groceries.

■ Take note of the kinds of food you eat that precipitate an attack. Eliminate them from your diet and re-introduce them slowly, one at a time once a week, to confirm what triggers the problem. Some people have lactose intolerance and react to milk products. Try eating fresh, unsweetened yoghurt made from cow's milk. Add a little roasted, coarsely

---

ADD NATURAL FIBRE TO YOUR DIET. EAT WHOLEGRAIN WHEAT FLOUR WITH ITS HUSK, OAT BRAN, VEGETABLES, COOKED BEANS, PULSES AND GUAR GUM. TOO MUCH FIBRE CAN SOMETIMES PRODUCE GAS, SO IF YOU ARE NOT USED TO IT, AND HAVE BEEN LIVING ON REFINED CARBOHYDRATES, INTRODUCE THESE SLOWLY. GIVE YOUR SYSTEM TIME TO ADJUST. WITH FIBRE YOU NEED TO DRINK A LOT OF FLUIDS, DO NOT HAVE IT JUST BEFORE OR AFTER YOUR MEAL. YOU ALSO NEED 6-7 GLASSES OF WATER A DAY.

pounded cummin seeds and a pinch of rock salt to your yoghurt.

■ Reduce fats in your diet, as fat stimulates colon contractions that worsen already irritable bowels.

■ Avoid coffee—there are some resins in the coffee bean other than caffeine which can cause the irritation.

■ Cut out smoking, red wine and beer from your diet.

AMOEBIASIS

Amoebiasis is a parasitic infection of the large intestine. It is a difficult infection to treat with allopathic drugs, and repeated courses of specific medication are needed.

Causes and symptoms

It is characterised by non-specific diarrhoea with loose, semi-formed, foul-smelling stools, or dysentery with mucous, traces of blood, and small quantities of stools passed repeatedly. Often there is an ineffectual urge to defecate again and again, with very little stool actually being passed. There is much flatulence, with abdominal cramps. In severe cases, the liver and other organs may get affected, causing specific conditions related to the organ, e.g., hepatitis, cysts, abscess, etc.

Remedies

■ Remove the kernel from the dried seeds of the *bael* fruit, and also the mango seed kernel. Take equal quantities of these two kernels. A teaspoonful of each kernel should be ground together. One-fourth of the mixture should be taken with a cup of rice gruel once a day for 3-4 days.

■ A once-a-week intake of ripe *bael* sherbat keeps the bowels in a healthy condition.

■ Roast unripe *bael* fruit on an open fire and remove its pulp. This should be eaten with a little jaggery or sugar—a teaspoonful daily is especially beneficial for blood diarrhoea with mucus.

■ Jam made with the semi-ripe or unripe *bael* fruit—a teaspoonful on an empty stomach every morning keeps the digestive system healthy.

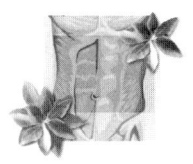

DIARRHOEA

The passage of repeated loose stools is called diarrhoea. It can be acute or chronic, and cause acute physical distress.

Causes and symptoms

Diarrhoea can be caused by dietary indiscretion, food intolerance, or a bacterial/viral infection of the gastro-intestinal tract. Sometimes anxiety and stress also play an important role. A change of place, travelling to new places, change of weather and water, may cause diarrhoea too.

It may also be associated with vomiting – a result of infection. Other complaints include headache, loss of appetite, nausea, pain in the abdomen, and a feeling of weakness and restlessness.

Remedies

■ Avoid solid food. Replace fluids and electrolytes lost in diarrhoea and vomiting by taking plenty of fluids, to avoid dehydration.

■ A simple oral rehydration fluid, which can be made at home, is to take a glass of boiled cooled water, and add a pinch of salt and a level teaspoon of sugar (you can replace this with jaggery) to it. Sip a glassful slowly. Have this after every loose motion. The total intake of fluid should be at least 6-7 glasses in a day. It is necessary to sip this and not gulp it down, because the sudden intake may trigger a bout of vomiting. This can be flavoured with fresh lime or fresh orange juice.

■ Grate an apple and leave it on a plate to brown. Mash and eat it slowly once a day.

■ Roast an unripe *bael* fruit over a coal fire. Remove the skin and collect the pulp. Take a teaspoon of this with warm water twice a day.

■ Grate a tender, unripe *bael* fruit after removing its skin. Dry, powder and store it. Take a teaspoon of this with warm water twice a day.

■ Make a paste of a teaspoon each of powdered cummin seeds, cinnamon and dry ginger with honey. Dissolve a teaspoonful in a cup of warm water and have it thrice a day.

- Boil a teaspoon of crushed cummin seeds in a cup of water for 2-3 minutes. Grind a tablespoon of washed, fresh coriander leaves. Add this to the cooled cummin herbal tea. Add a pinch of salt. Drink 2-3 times a day after a light meal of *khichri*.

- Shell a green cardamom pod and powder the seeds. Take half a teaspoonful of the powdered seeds and boil in a cup of water. Cool and drink cold, warm or hot, as desired, for chronic diarrhoea due to indigestion. Cardamom, however, is constipating.

- Take a small piece of the bark of a fig tree. Powder it. Add half a level teaspoon of the powdered bark to a teacup of fresh buttermilk. Have it once a day for chronic diarrhoea. Fig bark has carminative as well as astringent properties. It is especially useful for diarrhoea in children.

- Take equal quantities of dry ginger powder and fennel powder. A teaspoon of this, mixed with tea, or made into a herbal tea, flavoured with honey to taste – a cupful 3-4 times a day—is very effective.

- Powder a handful of dried mango flowers. This can be stored in powder form. Take a teaspoon of this powder with a teaspoon of honey once a day.

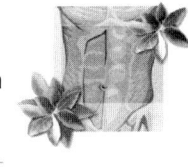

- Remove the kernel from 2-3 jambul seeds and a mango seed. Grind a teaspoon of each to a paste, and add to a glass of fresh buttermilk. Have it once a day. Both these kernels have astringent properties and are traditionally used for chronic diarrhoea.

- Take a tablespoon of the pounded bark of the jambul tree. Boil it in a glass of water to make a decoction till one-fourth of a glass remains. Filter and cool. A tablespoon of this decoction, mixed with a tablespoon of goat's milk, is used to control diarrhoea. The bark has astringent properties.

- Take 8-10 tender jambul leaves or leaf buds. Grind them with a little water. Then add a glass of water and stir well. Filter and drink with a teaspoon of honey.

- Take a lotus flower rhizome, the 'stem', which is inside the water. Cut it into small bits and roast it over a coal fire till it is burnt. Now grind these burnt pieces. Take three teaspoons of this ash, mixed with a level teaspoon of cooking soda, mix it with thick buttermilk and drink it. The ash has binding as well as moisture-soaking properties. It thickens and binds the stool. Combining with soda, the mixture reduces the gases formed in the intestine. The rhizome has starches with an arrowroot-like nutrient valve. So all the constituent have a multi-pronged effect and set the diarrhoea right.

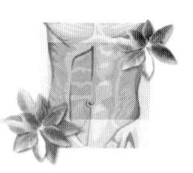

■ Summer diarrhoeas are usually self-limiting and need fluid replacement more than medicine. Drinking ORS (oral rehydrating solution) and eating the fresh, tender kernels of water chestnuts, known as *shinghara*, either fresh, boiled or roasted, with buttermilk, provides nourishment as well as fluid and minerals. This too has a binding action.

■ Take a teaspoon of the dry powdered bark of the banyan tree. Make an infusion using a glass of hot water. Let it steep for a while. This water is 'cooling' and helps control diarrhoea. Take half a glass of this infusion twice a day

■ Mix less than one-sixth of a teaspoon of powdered nutmeg in a tablespoon of hot water, add it to a glass of buttermilk and drink it. It decreases the motility of the intestine, and helps control a 'running tummy.' Too much of it however, can cause severe constipation. Hence, do not have it more than once a day for two days.

■ Unripe banana: Boil an uripe banana with the skin on. Let it simmer for 3-4 minutes on a low fire. Remove the skin of the banana and slice it. Heat two teaspoons of ghee in a vessel, splutter 2-3 cloves and add the sliced banana. Add one-fourth of a teaspoon of turmeric, one-fourth to half a teaspoon of rock salt, half a teaspoon of ground coriander seeds, and a tablespoon of yoghurt, or a cup of buttermilk. Cover and cook for a while. The unripe plantain or banana is astringent and antibilious.

■ Mash a tender, just ready to eat banana (not over-ripe) and have with a cup of milk twice a day. It useful in diarrhoea and dysentery.

■ Slice a tender, just ready-to-eat plantain, sprinkle rock salt on it for taste and smear half a tablespoon of tamarind pulp on it. Mix and have it twice a day.

■ Banana flower juice: Two tablespoons of fresh banana flower juice, mixed with a cup of buttermilk, taken twice a day, thickens stools and controls diarrhoea.

■ Crush a handful of fresh curry leaves. Grind them to a paste. Add one-fourth of a cup of water. Strain and have this curry-leaf juice with a teaspoon of honey once or twice a day. Chewing a few curry leaves twice a day will also help.

- Fresh mint juice: A tablespoonful with a few drops of fresh lime juice and honey is a good digestive and also soothing for chronic diarrhoea. This can be taken 2-3 times a day.

- Similarly, a teaspoon of the juice of fresh drumstick leaves, taken with fresh tender coconut water, replenishes fluids, vitamin-C and electrolytes.

- Slice a ripe banana lengthwise. Sprinkle one-eighth of a teaspoon of powdered nutmeg on the cut surface. Put both slices together and eat it. Do not repeat. Have it only once.

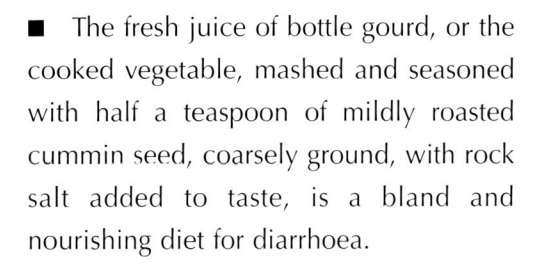

- Have one-fourth of a cup of pomegranate juice 2-3 times a day.

- The fresh juice of bottle gourd, or the cooked vegetable, mashed and seasoned with half a teaspoon of mildly roasted cummin seed, coarsely ground, with rock salt added to taste, is a bland and nourishing diet for diarrhoea.

- Carrot soup: Boil and mash half a kilogram of pealed, cubed carrots. Take a tablespoon of this pulp, mix it with half a cup of water and a little rock salt

---

THE DIET FOR DIARRHOEA PATIENTS SHOULD BE LIGHT, E.G., SPLIT MUNG DAL AND RICE *KHICHRI* SEASONED WITH CUMMIN SEEDS, WITH ROCK SALT ADDED FOR TASTE. BUTTERMILK IS SOOTHING AND REPLENISHING. POMEGRANATE JUICE, GINGER JUICE, COOKED, UNRIPE PLANTAINS AND BITTER GOURD ARE ALSO GOOD. AVOID LEAFY VEGETABLES, WHOLEGRAIN WHEAT OR PULSES, GARLIC, CUCUMBER, FRIED AND SPICY FOOD, ALCOHOL, ETC.

DIARRHOEA LEADS TO POTASSIUM DEPLETION. *BAEL* FRUIT IS RICH IN POTASSIUM AND ENSURES THAT THE CORRECT LEVEL IS MAINTAINED IN THE SOFT TISSUES BY PROPERLY BALANCING ELECTROLYTES INSIDE AND OUTSIDE THE INDIVIDUAL CELLS.

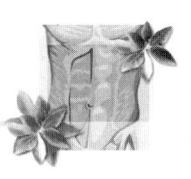

to taste, and have it 4-6 times a day. This does no harm at all. It can be taken more often if desired. It prevents putrefaction in the intestine and helps the healing process.

■ Boil a tablespoon of pounded peepul-tree bark with a glass of water, till half remains. Filter and take a teaspoon of this filtrate. Add just a small pinch of nutmeg powder and a glass of buttermilk. Drink this 2-3 times a day. The nutmeg powder should be less than a pinchful, not more. Take only for a day.

■ Infusion of rose petals: Add a tablespoon of crushed rose petals to a cup of boiling water. Filter and drink twice a day.

■ Take 4-5 soft, fresh, new leaf-buds from an Indian gooseberry shrub. Grind to a fine paste. Add to a cupful of fresh buttermilk, and drink twice or thrice a day.

■ A teaspoon of fenugreek seeds, soaked for half an hour in just enough water, then fried in a little butter, should be added to fresh buttermilk. A cupful drunk twice a day allays biliousness and rumbling in the stomach.

DYSENTERY

Dysentery is a disorder of the large intestines caused by pathogenic organisms. In this condition there is the constant urge to pass stool.

Causes and symptoms

In dysentery, there is not much diarrhoea, but mostly mucus and blood with a little faecal matter. There is ulceration in the large intestine which accounts for this constant irritability of the colon. The urge to pass stools is preceded by pain and tenesmus. A slight amount of stool and the slough of the ulcers pass as mucus and blood. Dysentery can be acute or chronic depending on the intensity of the complaints. Sometimes there is the passage of hard stools with a lot of mucus. Acute cases often come down with fever. According to modern medicine the cause of dysentery is microbial, whereas ayurveda, which is a way of healthy living, states that dietary indiscretions, climatic changes, wrong foods, incompatible dietary combinations, a hurried way of life, and an unhealthy environment, makes a substrate for these microbial infections to take root in susceptible people.

Remedies

All the remedies for diarrhoea will also come in handy here.

■ At the start of the problem, if a herbal decoction is made with two tablespoons of dried coriander seeds, and taken with plain water or buttermilk, the intestinal lining is soothed, and the quantity of mucus in the stool decreases.

■ The *bael* fruit remedy given in the diarrhoea section is also useful here. An unripe *bael* fruit should be roasted on a coal fire, the peel removed, and the pulp taken out. A tablespoon of this pulp should be taken 3-4 times a day with a glass of buttermilk, or plain, boiled, cooled water, with enough jaggery to sweeten it, and half a teaspoon of ginger juice, to give it a tang, as well as for the medicinal benefit of ginger. Unripe *bael* pulp has astringent properties.

■ Fresh lemon juice: Have the juice of two lemons added to a glass of water, with rock salt and sugar to taste, 3-4 times a day.

■ Take a tablespoon of dried orange peel, crushed and ground to a powder. Add a tablespoon of large black raisin seeds. The fruit part of the raisin is laxative in nature, whereas the seeds are not. Powder the seeds, and add it to the crushed, powdered, dried orange peel. Take a teaspoon of this mixture once a day for 3-4 days. The combination heals the ulcers in the intestines and stops the passage of mucus in stools

■ Take a tablespoon each of fresh mango flowers and pomegranate flowers. Mango flowers are small and grow in bunches on the tree, whereas pomegranate flowers are bigger, hence just one or two of them will suffice. Grind them together and mix in a glass of buttermilk. Both have astringent as well as soothing properties. The mango flower also has a styptic action which will stop the oozing of blood. Hence, both these act on the ulcers in the intestine. Have once a day for 3-4 days.

■ Take a tablespoon of fenugreek seeds. Grind and keep aside. One-fourth of a teaspoon of this powder, with a cup of fresh yoghurt, had 2-3 times a day, clears the mucus in the stool. Alternatively, a tablespoon of the juice of fenugreek leaves, taken with

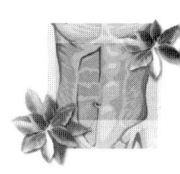

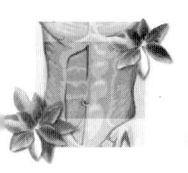

1-2 black raisins, will also relieve dysentery.

- In dysentery, where only blood and mucus is being passed, and instead of diarrhoea there are constipated stools, a teaspoon of dry ginger powder, mixed in a glass of hot water or hot milk, with a tablespoon of castor oil, will clear the intestines of blockage, quickly lubricating the lining. Follow this after a day or two with a teaspoon of psyllium hust powder in half a cup of yoghurt, taken twice a day for 3-4 days.

Note: *All the remedies given above replace fluids, electrolytes, trace elements and also the natural flora of the intestine, thereby ensuring a holistic approach to healing.*

GASTRO ENTERITIS / FOOD POISONING

Stop solid foods for 24 hours. Replace the fluids lost and slowly introduce soft, digestible meals. The remedies listed for diarrhoea will all come in handy here.

CHOLERA

Cholera is a condition that occurs very often in summer or in the rainy season in many parts of India. This is an acute intestinal infection, the sudden onset of which is characterised by excessive vomiting and the passage of several watery stools. This lethal combination leads to rapid dehydration, and circulatory collapse with a fatal outcome. The transmission is man-to-man by the oro-faecal route, spread by flies and unhygienic living conditions. The infection is so rapid that it can spread within a few hours to a few days from when the first cases begin to occur. The passage of motions may be 6-10 within an hour, with fever and projectile vomiting. Initially, the diarrhoea is painless, but soon abdominal cramps begin because of rapid dehydration and electrolytes lost. The eyes have a sunken look, the tongue becomes dry, and urinary output diminishes.

Timely help is the essence of the treatment. Cholera is a life-threatening disease and the fluid loss is so rapid that no chances can or should be taken. It is best to take the patient to a hospital for intravenous fluids and antibiotics. However, when that is not possible, the following remedies could help.

Remedies

■ Onion juice is considered especially useful in folk medicine. A teaspoon of onion juice added to a teaspoon of neem-fruit pulp (neem fruit grows during the cholera-prone months)should be licked from the spoon every 30 minutes or so. Two spoonsful last about two hours. The combination is very bitter, but it is not possible to mix it with water as that will cause the patient to vomit. However, just taking a lick and sipping water makes the patient feel better and changes the taste in the mouth. Besides, both these have antiseptic and anti-microbial properties that annihilate the cholera bacteria and also neutralise the toxin it liberates.

■ Grind 2-4 neem leaves with 3-4 black peppercorns and give the patient this mixture in a cupful of water, to sip slowly. Both these have anti-microbial properties.

■ Grind 6-8 holy basil and 6-8 neem leaves with a pinch of asafoetida powder. Roll it into a small pill with jaggery. This should be given 3-4 times a day.

■ Grind 4-5 cloves and mix with a pinch of asafoetida and jaggery. Have it 2-3 times with water.

■ Grind 5-6 black peppercorns into a paste with a medium-sized onion. Divide this chutney into four portions. Have it four times a day with a little water. Mashed onion is antimicrobial and allays thirst and restlessness.

■ Tender coconut water is an ideal rehydrating and nourishing drink with a teaspoon of fresh drumstick-leaf juice and a spoonful of honey added to it.

■ One-eight of a teaspoon of nutmeg powder, infused in a glass of water, cooled, mixed with the same amount of coconut water, and half a cupful of this drink taken every half an hour, will reduce the severity of the symptoms.

■ Clove-water decoction: Grind half a tablespoon of cloves. Boil it in two litres of water till it is reduced to a litre. Filter, cool and have this many times a day.

■ Celery-leaf infusion: Take a handful of celery leaves and grind them to a paste. Boil them in one-and-a half litres of water till only half remains. Give a spoonful of this cooled decoction every 15-20 minutes, till the patient's stool begins to thicken. Once that happens, stop this treatment. The natural restorative process would have begun. However, continue to give oral rehydration fluids

JAUNDICE / HEPATITIS

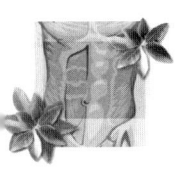

The yellowing of the whites of the eyes, the mucous membranes of the body and the skin due to an underlying liver dysfunction or disorder is called jaundice.

Causes and symptoms

Jaundice is caused by an accumulation of bile products. It could also be due to the blockage of the bile duct, infection or inflammation, or toxic damage to the liver cells. This infection/ inflammation of the liver is called hepatitis. Hepatitis is often caused by a viral infection of the liver, passed by the oro–faecal route, i.e., contaminated food or water, or through infected blood or blood products via contaminated needles. Untreated hepatitis leads to cirrhosis of the liver, irreversible liver damage, even cancer and death.

Other than yellowing of the skin, the symptoms include loss of appetite, fever, nausea, vomiting, severe fatigue, vague pains in the abdomen and headache.

Remedies

- Have plenty of fresh sugar cane juice to which the juice of a fresh lime and one-fourth of a teaspoon of rock salt has been added. The juice must be prepared fresh and the source checked for its cleanliness. This can be had 3-4 times, but in small amounts. The body's defence mechanisms are at a low ebb in hepatitis, so one must be careful in treating it gently, and not inadvertently causing diarrhoea.

- Lemon juice with sugar can be taken often.

- Fresh radish-leaf juice: Radish leaves are a lesser-known remedy for jaundice. A cupful of this juice in divided doses should be given throughout the day. Continue treatment for 3-4 days. The total intake should not to exceed a glassful, i.e, 250 ml.

- To make a snake gourd-leaf and coriander-seed infusion, add a tablespoon of pounded coriander seeds to a glass of hot water. Keep aside for half an hour. Cool and filter. Simultaneously, make an infusion of fresh snake gourd leaves. Mix two tablespoons of crushed leaves to two glasses of water. Boil and simmer for 4-5 minutes. Cool and filter. Mix both the filtrates and give the patient half a cup 3-4 times a day.

- Split red gram leaves: The leaves of this plant have a marked effect on liver function. Presumably they have some alkaloids which effect enzymatic activity. (Traditionally, farming was a rural occupation but lately a number of well-to-do city folk have also taken to farming in a big way. This information is for those who cultivate this crop but may not be aware of this nugget of knowledge in the era of hepatitis-A, B, C, and as yet undiagnosed variants!) Antiviral drugs are prohibitably expensive, and as yet no sure allopathic cure for hepatitis has been found.

Take a handful of the leaves and grind them to a paste. Add half a glass of boiled, cooled water. Leave aside for a while. Filter and drink the filtrate—a tablespoon thrice a day.

- Similarly, the juice extracted from fresh *bael*-tree leaves has a particularly beneficial effect. Eight to ten fresh leaves, ground to a fine paste, with a pinch of black pepper powder mixed with a glassful of buttermilk, taken thrice a day, is an effective remedy for jaundice.

- Half a teaspoon of the paste of fresh, tender papaya leaves enriches liver enzymes because of its rich B-carotene content, which helps damaged liver cells to heal. This can be taken with water twice a day.

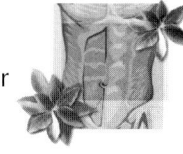

- Turmeric has antiseptic as well as healing properties. One-fourth of a teaspoon of turmeric stirred in a glass of warm water, taken thrice a day with a little jaggery, is beneficial.

- Half a teaspoon of turmeric can be added to a cup of fresh yoghurt or buttermilk and drunk thrice a day.

- The all-complete natural food, banana: Mash or slice a ripe banana. Lace it with honey and eat it twice a day—an excellent antidote.

- Indian gooseberry chutney or sherbet with jaggery, taken 3-4 times a day, is nourishing for the liver. For the chutney, crush 1-2 fresh Indian gooseberries into a paste with jaggery. Lick the paste and drink a glass of water after licking it, or stir

N HEPATITIS OR JAUNDICE DUE TO ANY CAUSE, FIRST STOP ALL FATS IN THE DIET. AVOID REFINED CARBOHYDRATES, I.E., WHITE FLOUR PRODUCTS, FRIED FOODS AND ALCOHOL. HAVE A SIMPLE, EASILY DIGESTABLE LIGHT CARBOHYDRATE DIET.

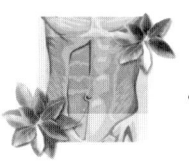

a spoonful into a glass of water and drink it 2-3 times a day.

■ Fresh mint juice with ginger, lime and honey often allays biliousness in jaundice and stimulates the appetite.

Note: *A smaller version of the lemon-sized Indian gooseberry is* phyllanthus amarus. *These fruits are the size of mung dal. Any part of this plant is useful in jaundice. Grind 2-3 fruits to a paste. Add a teaspoon of this to a glass of buttermilk .Have 2-3 times a day for 10 days This has been found effective in all types of hepatitis. Many recent studies have validated these findings.*

GALLSTONES

Gallstones are a collection of normal or abnormal bile constituents in the gall bladder which cause excrutiating pain.

Causes and symptoms

Cholesterol, which is a lipid processed from the intake of fats present in the food, is a water-insoluble substance. The addition of bile, which is produced by the liver and stored in the gall bladder, enters the intestine via the bile duct and interacts with the cholesterol to make it soluble. If this cholesterol does not dissolve, it gets precipitated and is deposited in the gall bladder as concretions of cholesterol, bile pigments, calcium and other constituents. These are gallstones, which are stones of different types, depending on their composition.

Gallstones may be single or multiple. They cause pain when they either block the bile duct, or are so many that they stretch the gall bladder wall.

Remedies

■ Have a fat-free diet.

■ Have a diet rich in artichokes—globe artichokes. These have a substance called cynarin, which helps control cholesterol levels and improves liver and gall bladder function.

■ Beetroots and beetroot juice are especially beneficial as they clean the gall bladder. The juice can be combined with carrot juice, both in equal quantities. Take half a cup of each. Mix and have it twice a day.

■ Among fruits, pears has a positive effect on gall bladder function.

PILES/ANAL FISSURE

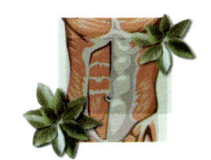

Swollen and protruding veins in and around the anus are known as piles. The veins that drain the blood from the tissues in the anal area lie at the junction of the rectum and the anus. The rectum is the last part of the large intestine or colon, and the anus is the external aperture at the end of the gastrointestinal canal, through which the waste products are finally expelled as faeces or stools. The venous drainage of this area is just inside the anal opening.

Causes and symptoms

When there is straining during defecation, the muscles of this area contract and put pressure on the veins. If the valves in the wall of the veins are weak, there is engorgement of blood in the veins, causing them to protrude. This engorgement of veins is also called varicose veins. The engorged protruding veins that lie external to the anal orifice are called external piles, and these can be felt. The veins that lie internal to the orifice cannot be seen or felt normally. Constipation is one of the main causes of piles, but any systematic disorder involving the liver, e.g., cirrhosis, or back pressure in the circulation due to any cause, a prostate enlargement, pregnancy, chronic coughing, etc., can all cause pressure in the venous drainage in this area.

People only become aware of piles when they bleed or there is pain. Initially, piles do not hurt. That only happens when infection sets in. So do not neglect any bleeding from the anus, however slight it may be. Bleeding may be the first sign of cancer of the colon. Sometimes, because of the engorgement, there may be a little mucus discharge. This causes itching, which is when a person should visit the doctor to find out the cause.

Sometimes there are no symptoms of piles (if the veins in the area are normal), and there is no systematic cause for pressure in the area. However, the passage of hard, constipated stools cause trauma to the anal orifice, and a linear ulcer occurs. Trauma due to any cause—anal intercourse, a particularly traumatic childbirth, or post-operative lesions—can result in a linear cut, forming an ulcer. This is called an anal fissure. Anal fissures cause a sharp agonising pain during defecation, and they set up a vicious cycle of constipation. If constipation is the cause of the fissure, and the fissure is painful, a person avoids passing motions, which then results in him or her not responding to the call of nature and getting more constipated. All in all, most gastrointestinal de-arrangements are only the result of the bowels not being cleared regularly. This may be a hereditary disorder, where there is a congenital weakness of the veins in this area, in which case, more than one person in the family will present with piles, and at an earlier age.

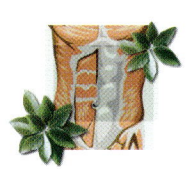

All remedies for constipation will ease the problem. But diarrhoea, when it is the result of overuse of laxatives, will result in a fissure becoming inflamed and painful.

Remedies

Neem and holy basil head the list of remedies for piles in folk medicine.

- Powder a measure each of dried neem seeds and the roots of the holy basil plant (which has been washed and dried). This can be stored in a dry container. A level teaspoon of this mixture, taken once a day with a glass of buttermilk for 2-3 weeks, heals piles. Neem seeds have a laxative as well as emollient action. Holy basil leaves are digestive and styptic, i.e., they stop bleeding. Between the two, they put liver function right (unless there is an inherent weakness in the veins), and help clean the bowels regularly, controlling the oozing of blood at the site. Both have antimicrobial and antiseptic properties. Holy basil leaves also have an anti-inflammatory, analgesic action. They relieve pain. This preparation also heals fissures.

- For bleeding piles: A teaspoonful of black sesame seeds, ground to a paste and taken with half a glass of goat's milk, to which a teaspoon of jaggery is added, will clear the bleeding and discomfort of piles in two days. Have once a day for 2-3 days.

- A teaspoon of black sesame seeds, ground to a paste, with a little jaggery and butter added, taken twice a day for a week, heals piles. Sesame seeds have a laxative action. The paste also has emollient properties, and so it soothes and heals the passage. The medicament in the paste tones up the blood vessels in the area.

- A decoction of sesame seeds is just as beneficial. Pound coarsely a tablespoon of seeds and boil them in half a litre of water till only a glassful remains. This should be kept aside. Have one-fourth of a glass twice a day.

- The peel of a pomegranate, boiled in a glass of water, cooled and filtered and drunk once a day, is soothing for piles.

COCONUT

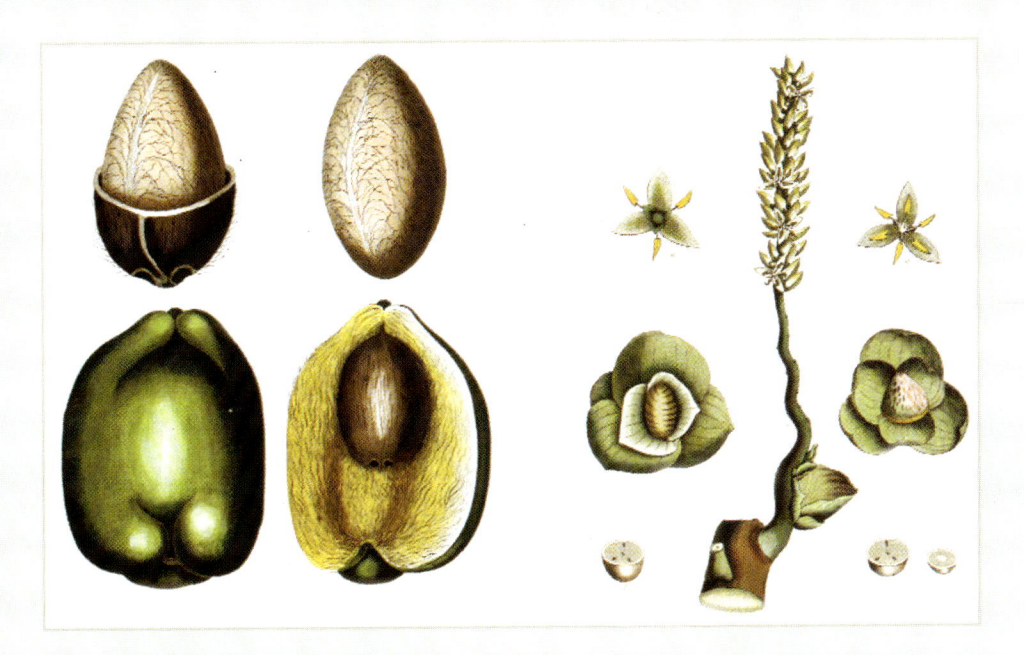

Botanical name: *Cocos nucifera*

Description and uses: The coconut is the large, ovate brown seed of the coconut palm. It has a fibrous husk around a hard shell lined with edible white flesh, which encloses a cloudy, almost transparent liquid.

Coconut oil/paste and milk extracted from coconut flesh, as well as tender coconut water, are effectively used to treat problems related to the head, anaemia, hypertension, chapped lips, toothache, indigestion, dyspepsia, biliousness, diarrhoea, cholera, intestinal worms, a burning sensation or pain during urination, an increase in the frequency of urination, arthritis, muscle strains and sprains, nappy rash, boils, white patches on the skin, blackheads, eczema, pruritis, hair problems, corns, calluses and rough heels.

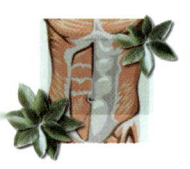

- Mix half a teaspoon of ginger juice, a teaspoon of fresh lime juice, a pinch each of rock salt, black pepper powder, long pepper powder, a tablespoon each of fresh mint juice and honey, and dissolve them in a glass of buttermilk or plain water. Have it once a day. It is helpful in healing piles.

- Juice of onion: A tablespoon with a little ghee and sugar should be taken twice a day for a few days.

- The juice of bitter gourd leaves is very beneficial. Two or three teaspoons of the fresh juice of the leaves with a glass of buttermilk should be drunk once a day.

- Radishes and turnips are root vegetables which should be eaten as a salad daily as a treatment for piles.

- Dried mango-seed powder: One fourth of a teaspoon of the powder, with the same amount of honey, should be taken twice a day. Mango seeds can be collected in season, dried and powdered, and the powder stored. It has many uses. What is available in the market is unripe mango-peel powder, which many housewives buy as a spice to use in cooking. This is not the same as mango-seed powder.

For local application on painful piles or fissures-in-ano

- Neem and holy basil leaves, ground together and made into a paste, can be applied as a poultice.

- Neem-seed oil should be applied locally.

- Sometimes a cool application gives more relief. Take a tablespoon of sesame seed, a tablespoon of crushed neem leaves, and a 2-inch stick of liquorice. Grind them to a paste with milk. Apply locally on the piles / fissure.

- Roasted onion, mashed and placed in a cloth and applied as a poultice while still warm, is highly efficacious.

INTESTINAL WORMS

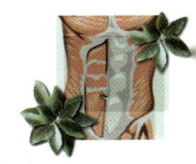

The digestive tract can be infested with many types of parasites or worms which can cause health problems of great magnitude.

Causes and symptoms

Parasites or worms are caused by the ingestion of contaminated food, eating uncooked infected meat, or vegetable/salads which have not been properly washed in clean water. Of these, threadworms, pinworms and roundworms are very commonly seen in children.

The symptoms are loss of appetite, pain in the abdomen, diarrhoea, vomiting, unexplained rashes and cyclic episodes of cough (these bouts being more at night) which occur every 4-6 weeks. Tapeworm infection can form cysts in the brain, and a convulsion may be the first presenting symptom.

Remedies

■ Soak 3-4 crushed, fresh garlic cloves in one-fourth cup of milk at night. Next morning press the cloves, remove them and drink the filtrate.

■ Soak 8-10 crushed cloves of garlic in a cup of water overnight. Next morning use this water to give an enema. This is especially beneficial for pinworms.

■ Take a tablespoon of dry neem flowers. Fry them in a teaspoon of ghee and eat them with boiled rice twice a day for 3-4 days.

■ Have a teaspoon of dried neem-leaf powder with milk or hot water twice a day for a week.

■ Make a decoction of a tablespoon of powdered neem-tree bark with two

---

SPECIALLY FOR CHILDREN: Take a tablespoon of fresh neem flowers or tender, neem leaves, one-fourth of a teaspoon of omum, 2-3 black peppers, one-fourth teaspoon of fresh grated ginger, a teaspoon of fennel, with jaggery to taste. Grind all these together, fry in a teaspoon of oil and eat it with rice.

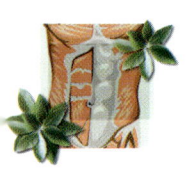

glasses of water and reduce it to half a glass. Two or three tablespoons of this should be taken twice a day for a week. Have it with milk or hot water.

- Remove the kernel of a dried mango seed and powder it. Half a tablespoon of this powder should be taken with thin buttermilk or water for two days.

- Powder 6-8 seeds bitter gourd seeds. Fry in a little ghee and have it twice a day for 3 or 4 days.

- Have a tablespoon of bitter gourd juice with a glass of buttermilk once a day for three days.

- Wash, dry and cut some banana-tree roots into pieces and burn them. One-fourth of this ash, taken with a teaspoon of honey for 4-7 days, will get rid of the worms.

- Collect a handful of pomegranate-root bark. Make a decoction with two glasses of water, with 4-5 crushed cloves added to it. Reduce it to half, and divide it into two doses. Filter, cool and drink it in the morning and evening. Next day, take any of the remedies mentioned in the section on constipation. In case the patient has been passing normal stools, a light laxative will do. If there is a tendency to constipation, take a remedy which will clear the bowels.

- Half a teaspoon of fenugreek seeds, fried and powdered, taken thrice a day for two days is efficacious.

- Powder 10-12 dried Indian gooseberries. Take a teaspoonful at bedtime on the first day. Thereafter, take a pinch in the morning and another in the evening for a week.

Unripe papaya has the digestive enzyme papain, which is toxic for worms, especially roundworms. Papaya leaves too are anti-helmintic. Soft, young papaya leaves or one leaf, as it is very large, can be used to make a decoction. Crush and dry one leaf. Powder it. Take a tablespoon of this crushed, dried, leaf powder and pour two glasses of boiling hot water over it. Leave it for an hour, and then filter and sweeten it with honey to taste. This can be taken in divided doses twice.

- Take a few seeds of the flame of the forest flower. Soak 2-3 teaspoons of these seeds in water for a couple of hours. Once the outer cover softens, remove it and extract the kernels. Dry, powder and store. Half a teaspoon of this powder, mixed with half teaspoon of dry Indian gooseberry powder, taken thrice a day for one day, removes intestinal parasites, especially roundworms and tapeworms. Mix 1-2 teaspoons of honey with it, as it is bitter to taste. Have for 2-3 days.

- Flame of the forest-seed kernel powder can also be taken by itself. Mix half a teaspoon of the powder with a teaspoon of honey, and drink it with warm water thrice a day for three days. On the fourth day, have a tablespoonful of castor oil, as a laxative, with a cup of milk, to expel the worms.

- Make a decoction of a handful of sliced drumsticks in two glasses of water, reduced to half a glass. Take a tablespoon of this decoction with a teaspoon of honey twice a day for one or two days.

- Pumpkin seeds: A level tablespoon of pumpkin seeds, crushed to a coarse powder, and taken with a cup of milk with a teaspoon of honey at bedtime for 3-5 days, gets rid of tapeworms.

- Have a tablespoon of crushed walnut kernel with a cup of hot water at bedtime for three days.

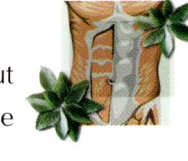

- Have a half a cup of fresh cabbage juice every morning for 3-5 days.

- Crush and powder 3-4 dried papaya seeds. Mix in a glass of warm milk and have every night for two days. Papaya seeds have a substance called carisin that destroys worms. Eating ripe papaya is also a healthy way to keep clear of worm infestation.

- Slice an unripe papaya and collect the juice. To a tablespoon of this juice, add a tablespoon of honey, and mix it in one-fourth to half a cup of boiling water. Cool it to an acceptable warmth and have it in one gulp as a draught. After one-and-a-half /two hours, take a tablespoonful of castor oil with a teaspoon of fresh lime juice. Some people may have colic or pain in the abdomen after this—have milk sweetened with honey or sugar. Children need to be given half or one-fourth of the dose for this remedy, as it is awful in taste and the castor oil causes purgation.

- Powdered betel nut: A level teaspoon, or a little less, taken with a glass of warm

SUGAR CANE

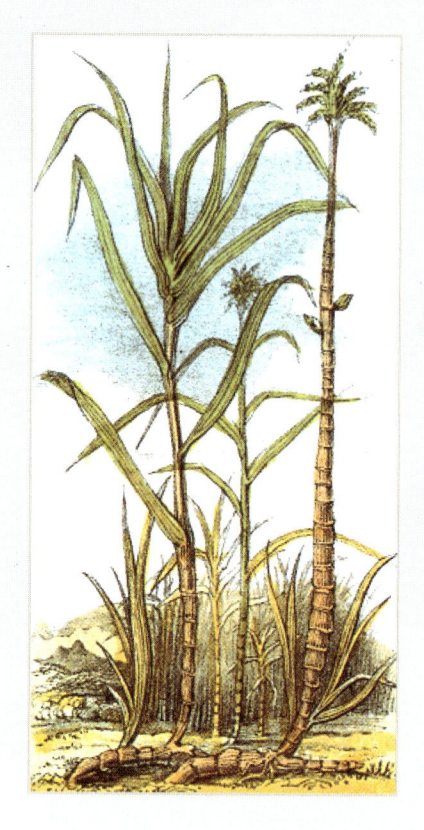

Botanical name: *Saccharum officinarum*

Description and uses: Sugar cane is a perennial tropical grass of the genus *saccharum*. It has tall, stout, jointed stems from which juice is extracted. This juice is used to make sugar. Apart from it being an important food element, sugar cane juice is highly efficacious for treating jaundice and hepatitis. In these ailments, where allopathic medicines have failed, sugar cane has proved to be an age-old, tried-and-tested remedy.

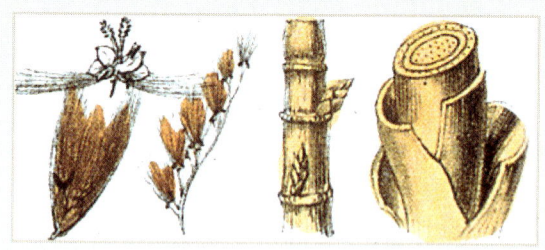

In half a cup of vinegar prepared from cane sugar/molasses, and not the artificial acetic acid one, soak a tablespoon of chickpeas overnight. Next morning eat the chickpeas after draining out the vinegar. Do not eat anything after that for 6-8 hours. Then you can have a meal.

milk on an empty stomach gets rid of tapeworms.

Remedies for Children

■ A tablespoon of radish juice taken twice a day with a pinch of rock salt for 4-5 days destroys intestinal worms.

■ One-eighth of a teaspoon of the dried pulp of the aloe leaf, taken with water at bedtime, is a potent purgative. This is very bitter, so the pulp can be ground with a little sugar and then had with water or apple juice.

■ Fasting and having only carrot juice for a day will also get rid of intestinal worms. For children it is not necessary to fast. But half a cup of carrot juice should be given every morning for three days. Do not give them any food for three hours after the juice.

■ Coconut is an important ingredient in South Indian cuisine. It also has its uses for getting rid of worms. A tablespoon of freshly ground coconut taken with a light breakfast, followed by two tablespoons of castor oil, and a glass of hot milk after four hours, will expel any worms in the intestine.

LOSS OF APPETITE

Loss of appetite, not wanting to eat, is a complaint related to many disorders. The underlying cause must be found and treated in all cases. However, to stimulate the appetite, the following are a few non-controversial remedies:

Remedies

■ Pound together a tablespoon each of dry ginger powder, dry black pepper powder, dry long pepper powder and rock salt powder. Mix. Take two cups of seedless, large dried black grapes. Grind them all together and store them in a glass container. Eat half a teaspoon of the mixture twice a day.

■ Fry two tablespoons of grated ginger in two tablespoons of ghee till it is a light brown in colour. Now add half a cup of jaggery powder and stir till the jaggery dissolves. Take it off the fire and store—half to one teaspoon, taken twice a day, stimulates the appetite.

Note: *All remedies listed under indigestion/heartburn will also stimulate the appetite.*

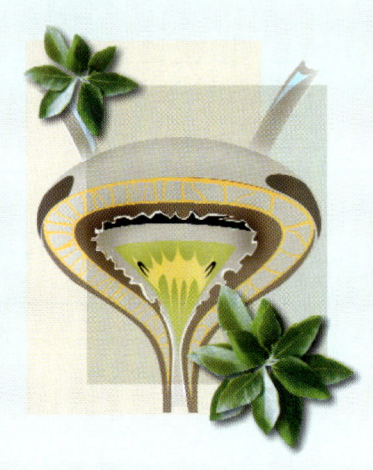

Our excretary organs are the kidneys, the ureters and the urinary bladder. There are several problems such as urinary-tract infections, blood in the urine, renal stones and prostrate-related complaints, which cause immense discomfort and distress, and need urgent remedial care.

URINARY COMPLAINTS

The kidneys, ureters and urinary bladder are our organs of excretion. They lie at the back of the abdomen on either side of the spine. The bladder lies in the pelvis, protected by the two hip bones. The kidneys filter the blood of its impurities and maintain the water and electrolyte balance in the body. Besides this, the kidneys also help in the regulation of blood pressure. Hence, any complaints related to this system will have far-reaching effects almost immediately. The main complaints related to the urinary system are the following:

A BURNING SENSATION IN PASSING URINE/PAIN WHILE PASSING URINE, AND AN INCREASE IN THE FREQUENCY OF PASSING URINE

Causes and symptoms

These complaints are usually suggestive of an urinary-tract infection. Urinary-tract infections are often bacterial in origin. They most frequently occur in young girls and women due to the inherent vulnerability of the anatomical placement of the urethra so close to the anus. Other causes may be renal stones, tumours, and non-specific infections of the urethra. But this is seldom so. Bacterial infection is the most common cause. Fever, chills, rigors and discomfort in the lower abdomen are the usual symptoms. Burning and pain at the urethral orifice, back pain, headache, nausea, vomiting, or even diarrhoea, may also occur. Very young children may only cry with pain while passing urine, unable to explain what they feel. However, failure to thrive, fever, vomiting and diarrhoea may be pointers to an underlying urinary-tract infection in young girls. In males, these complaints are uncommon after the age of one year, and they can again recur as related symptoms in prostrate enlargement or prostatitis after the age of 45 years. However, younger males with gonococcal infection—a venereal disease—will also have these complaints.

CELERY

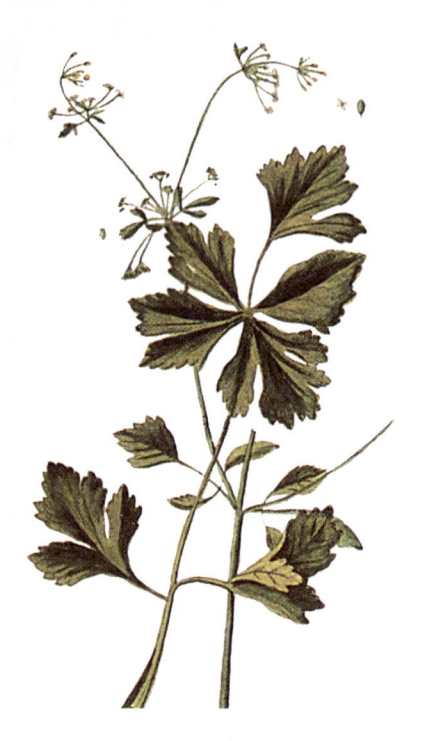

Botanical name: *Apium graveolens*

Description and uses: Celery is an umbelliferous plant with closely packed succulent leaf-stalks which are eaten as a vegetable. The parts used are the seeds, stalks and root. It has a characteristic, agreeable odour, and a warm, aromatic and slightly pungent teste. Celery has a carminative, stimulating and diuretic action. It is a tonic which is useful in hysteria, and promotes restfulness and sound sleep. It is also used to treat cholera, renal stones and arthritis.

Remedies

■ Drink plenty of water during the day to flush out the kidneys.

■ Fresh, green coconut water should be drunk daily 2-3 times .

■ Barley water: Boil a tablespoonful of barley in a glass of water. Make a watery gruel. You can thin it further by adding another glass of water, with salt and lime juice to taste. Have a glass of this 2-3 times a day.

■ Parsley herbal tea or infusion: Wash a handful of parsley leaves and crush them. Pour two glasses of boiling hot water over them. Cover and leave for 2-3 hours. Filter and drink it 2-3 times a day.

- Boil a teaspoon of grated lemon peel in a glassful of water. Have 2-3 times a day.

- Corn-silk tea/infusion: Don't throw away the silky tassels when you take off the leaves from a fresh corncob. Boil them in half a litre of water or make an infusion. It is excellent for flushing and toning up the kidneys.

- *Cynodon dactylon:* This is a common grass which grows in lawns. It is used as fodder for cattle. It has a long slender stem and grows as a runner, rooting at the nodes. It has branches and erect three-bladed leaves. The fruit is like a compressed grain. This grass needs to be washed very well. Grind a handful of fresh, thoroughly washed and cleaned grass with two small *phyllanthus amarus* to a fine paste. Stir into a glassful of diluted buttermilk. Divide it into two and drink this twice a day.

- Grated white pumpkin: To half a cupful, add a handful of washed *cynodon dactylon* and boil it with half a litre of water. Make a decoction. Drink one-third of a cup thrice a day. This is very good for genital-and urinary-tract infections.

- Have fresh carrot juice, half a cup, thrice a day.

- Jambul is excellent for urinary-tract infections. It contains anti-bacterial compounds called anthocyanins. These work against E-coli bacteria, which are the most common culprit in urinary-tract infections. They also have a substance which prevents bacteria from forming a nidus or sticking to the walls of the mucous membrane. Eating 8-10 jambul fruits every morning will keep the tract free of infection.

- Hibiscus flower infusion: Soak 8-10 flowers in one-and-a-half litres of water overnight. Drink two tablespoons 3-4 times a day for 2-3 days.

- Sandalwood: Grind a small flat piece of sandalwood in a circular motion on a flat marble stone with 2-3 drops of water. Half a teaspoon of this ground paste, mixed in a cup of milk and taken twice a day, helps clear urinary-tract infection. A pinch of powdered omum can also be added when the milk is being heated.

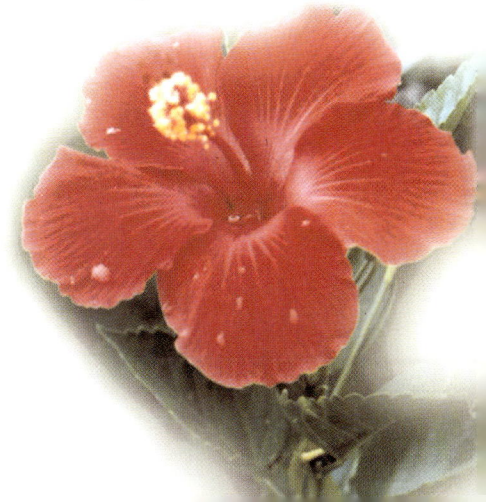

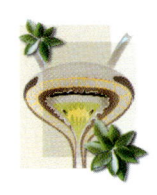

RENAL STONES

As mentioned earlier, the function of the kidneys is to maintain the water and electrolyte balance of the body. Electrolytes are composed of the calcium, sodium, potassium, magnesium, chloride, phosphate, sulphate and bicarbonate, etc., salts in the body. The kidneys conserve the amount of water needed and excrete the salts not required. This depends on the body's ability to adapt to changes in climate and diet, physical activity, and the inherent hormonal functions which affect calcium metabolism.

Causes and symptoms

In the summer months, due to a rise in environmental temperature and water losses due to perspiration, the concentration in solute increases. These urinary solutes have certain proteins that combine with calcium to form insoluble complexes that may result in the formation of a stone. However, nature has an in-built balancing mechanism in the form of certain citrates present in the urine that will help dissolve these insoluble complexes. But if there is hormonal imbalance, the urinary excretion of citrate decreases. This predisposes to stone formation. These hormones are female sex hormones. Female sex hormones fall during menstruation. Now, if there is superimposed urinary-tract infection, certain infective foci or nuclei form a nidus for the calcium to deposit around and form a stone. In this is involved another hormone, the parathyroid hormone, which regulates calcium metabolism. In the case of excessive secretion of this gland, excess calcium is excreted, which again predisposes to calculi formation. A deficiency of vitamin-A predisposes the mucous membrane of the tubules in the kidney to wear off much more easily. These cells, which are being shed, also form a nucleus, around which calcium deposits. To top this, if physical activity is low due to a sedentary lifestyle or recumbence due to illness. etc., there is stasis in the kidney, so once again sluggish circulation results in more time for calcium to be deposited.

The chemical composition of kidney stones may vary. You can only know what type of stones you have, in the event you pass one out and save it to get it analysed.

Seventy per cent of stones are calcium oxalate or calcium phosphate stones, and the ratio of occurrence is 3:1 as males to females. The age group is 40 – 50 years when you first become aware of them. Ten to fifteen per cent of these cases are due to hyperparathyroidism. Eight per cent of stones are due to infection – triple phosphate, calcium phosphate and magnesium ammonium phosphate stones. They are more common in women and occur in the childbearing years, i.e., 20 to 45 years. These stones are preventable and treatable, but untreated are a cause of renal failure.

Another eight per cent of stones are due to uric acid formation and occur more often in men after the age of 40 years. These are usually small like gravel. They are also radio translucent, may not always be seen on X-rays, and may need a CT scan for detection.

Cystine stones rarely occur in men and women who are below 25-30 years old. These are caused by a genetic autosomal recessive disease, where absorption of certain amino acids in the kidney tubules is faulty.

All stones do not cause symptoms. Phosphate stones may only be detected when they have really increased in size and have damaged renal tissue, causing blood in the urine.

Seventy-five per cent of patients with stones present with pain. The pain of a kidney stone is excruciating and depends on the site of the stone. A stone in the kidney will cause a pain in the lower back, just below the rib cage. This may radiate from the back to the front, into the loins. The pain is worse when there is movement. Stones that are small and have travelled into the ureters will cause pain in the loins. The patient doubles up with pain, and there may be frank blood in the urine. Sometimes a stone gets impacted in the urethra. The pain then radiates to the vulva in women and the tip of the penis in men. It is difficult to pass urine, and passing a drop causes sharp pain. However, stones which have reached the bladder may remain silent, causing no symptoms. Sometimes there is mild irritation inside the bladder that causes no pain, and the patient feels like emptying his bladder all the time. Pain only occurs when there is a jolting movement, e.g., a bumpy ride in a vehicle. Lying down diminishes the pain, while sitting upright again brings it on.

> IF YOU DO NOT HAVE A GENETIC PREDISPOSITION TO STONE FORMATION DUE TO INHERENT PHYSIOLOGICAL PROBLEMS, IN MOST CASES, TREATMENT CAN BE REGULATED BY DRINKING PLENTY OF FLUIDS, DIETARY MANAGEMENT AND ADEQUATE PHYSICAL ACTIVITY.

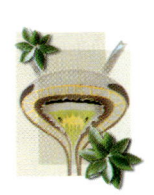

PUMPKIN SEEDS are known in folklore medicine for their efficacy in preserving the prostate gland and male potency. A daily dose of the kernel of the seeds – about a heaped tablespoon – chewed properly or pounded and mixed with cooked vegetables or chapattis is effective in getting rid of bladder complaints related to prostate enlargement, and also in containing the enlargement of the prostate. This prescription can also be had with milk and honey to taste. The seeds are rich in vitamin-E, which is considered an essential factor for the health of the prostate. Pumpkin seeds are also rich in zinc, which is vital for prostate function. Studies have shown that deficiency of zinc is related to an enlarged prostate. Prostate enlargement is caused by the build-up of di hydro testosterone, an intermediary product in the metabolism/formation of the male hormone testosterone. Zinc helps to contain this build-up. Studies have shown that patients with an enlarged prostate have low zinc levels. Zinc is found in plenty in nuts, seeds, whole grains, meat and shellfish – but the highest content is in pumpkin seed!

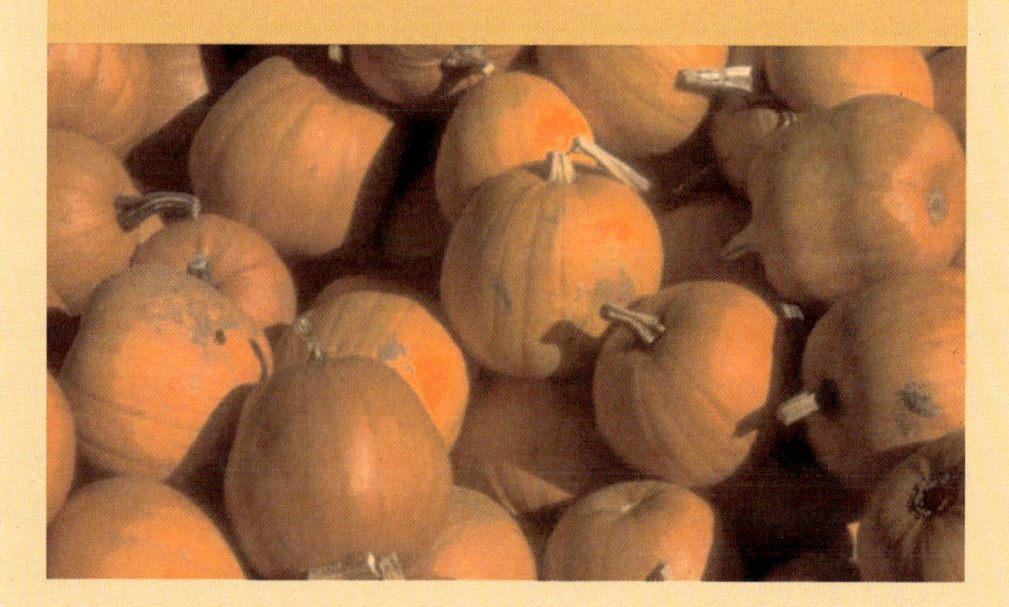

Remedies

Once it has been diagnosed, constant management and supervision is needed to avoid recurrence of stone formation. Drink plenty of fluids, especially water.

- Exercise moderately, like walking, riding a bike, etc.

- Go slow on calcium-rich foods. Do not eliminate them completely but restrict your intake of milk and dairy products.

- Cut out on oxalate-laden food, e.g., beets, beans, jambul, green peppers, parsley, spinach, strawberries, etc.

- Restrict your high-protein intake, such as meat, poultry, fish, etc.

- Increase your vitamin-A intake, but do not overload the system

- Holy basil is excellent for relieving kidney problems as well as for helping to expel stones. A teaspoonful of holy basil juice, with a teaspoon of honey in a glass of water, taken daily for 2-3 months, will help dissolve and expel the stone.

- Celery water or celery soup taken daily prevents stone formation in those prone to kidney stones.

- Three to four figs, boiled with a teacupful of water, should be taken daily for a month. The figs too should be eaten.

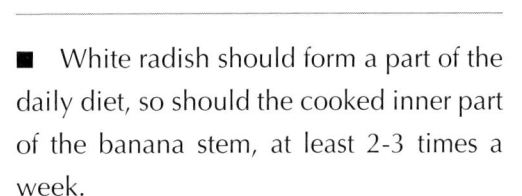

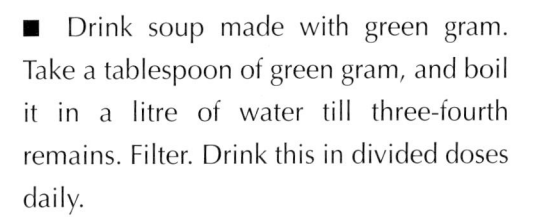

- White radish should form a part of the daily diet, so should the cooked inner part of the banana stem, at least 2-3 times a week.

- Drink soup made with green gram. Take a tablespoon of green gram, and boil it in a litre of water till three-fourth remains. Filter. Drink this in divided doses daily.

- Take a tablespoon of linseed. Crush them and boil them in a litre of water till three-fourth remains. Filter and add a teaspoon each of lemon juice and honey. Drink this 2-3 times a day. It is also very useful in cystitis, ie., inflammation of the urinary bladder.

- Parsley tea or parsley juice: Take a handful of washed parsley. Place in a dish and pour a litre of boiling water over it. Cover, let it cool and filter it. Drink it in divided doses. Take daily for 2-3 weeks. However, this remedy is not advisable for those with suspected oxalate stones.

- A decoction of barley is also good for flushing the kidneys out.

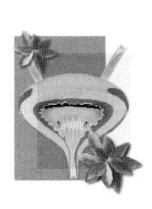

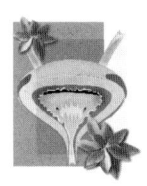

- Cantaloupe: The root, washed well, ground fine with water, strained, and a tablespoonful of this drunk daily in the early morning for seven days dissolves renal stones. Melon seeds, ground to a paste with water, and one-and-a-half teaspoonful taken daily in the early morning for seven days, have a similar action. This also clears other harmful deposits in the urine. However, this can only be done when fresh melons are available. The ripe fruit is green with a yellow tinge, and the lines on it are white.

RETENTION OF URINE AND PROSTATE RELATED-COMPLAINTS

The prostate is an organ of the male reproductive system. It is a firm glandular structure, and lies at the base of the urinary bladder at the beginning of the urethra. It secretes a fluid in which the sperms are suspended.

Causes and symptoms

Infection in the prostate can be caused by any retrograde infection from the urethra, or from a distant focus in the body, when it is blood borne. Prostate infection is called prostatitis, and presents with fever, chills, rigors, backache, lassitude and fatigue. There may be pain on passing urine and also pain during defecation. In some cases, there may be pain radiating to the back of the legs, fluid being passed from the urethra, premature ejaculation and temporary impotency. Prostate enlargement is a problem of 'menopausal' men. It occurs after the age of 50, and is a result of a decrease in androgenic hormones, which creates an imbalance with the oestrogenic female hormones. Males too have both the male and female hormones, but a balance is maintained throughout the reproductive phase for optimum 'male function'. When the prostate enlarges, it may project into the urinary bladder, its lobes may press on the urethra or the internal urethral orifice, causing the symptoms of increased frequency of urination, and the patient may need to get up often at night to pass urine. This problem becomes progressive. Urine is not passed in one go. Some residual urine remains, so the patient needs to pass it again and again. There is dribbling at the end of the act. This retention causes stasis and stagnation, so infection takes place. Because the bladder is distended most of the time, there is pain in the lower abdomen and lower back. Usually this enlargement is benign, but at times malignant changes occur.

Remedies

A surgeon must check up prostate-related complaints. However, some home remedies will relieve the symptoms.

■ Research in Germany has shown that the roots of stinging nettles (*urtica dioica*) yield a substance that relieves some of the symptoms of an enlarged prostate. If stinging nettles touch your skin, a violent itch and rash appears. Growing close to it is a type of spinach, and the juice of its crushed leaves, if applied immediately (even rubbing crushed leaves on the rash helps), will give relief. Boil a handful of the roots of stinging nettles in one-and-a half litres of water for 8-10 minutes, cool, filter it and drink half a cupful every 4-6 hours. It causes diuresis – urine begins to flow comfortably. It is also used to soothe and cure the irritation of an inflamed bladder with kidney stones.

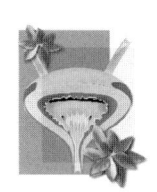

BLOOD IN THE URINE

Urine that is red in colour may not always mean that there is blood in it. Beetroot, vegetable dyes used in processed foods, or certain medicines can also cause its colour to be red.

Causes and symptoms

However, frank blood in urine is an alarming symptom and needs prompt and expert medical attention. The causes could be renal stones, which are easier to treat than renal cancer, which presents a more morbid scenario.

Blood in the urine is called haematuria, and this should never be treated at home. However, the remedies given below can be complementary to more orthodox treatment.

Remedies

■ Eat bitter gourd, unripe banana or plantain and drumsticks every day.

■ A tablespoon each of *phyllanthus amarus* juice and *cynodon dactylon* juice, added to a cup of fresh buttermilk, should be taken once a day. *Phyllanthus amarus* juice, or a tablespoon of the berry made into a paste and mixed with buttermilk, is also very beneficial.

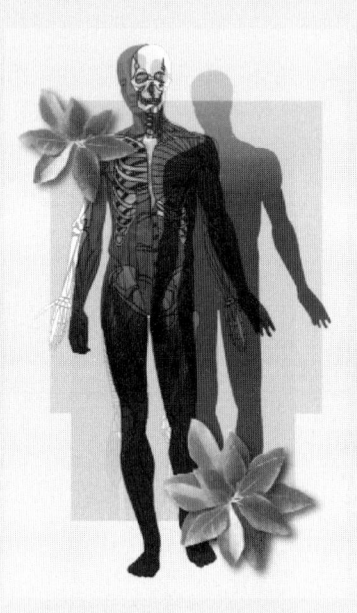

Our bones and muscles form the framework and support system which enclose all the vital organs in our body and also help us maintain our balance, sit, stand, lie down, run, walk, and so forth. Ailments such as arthritis, sciatica, backache, muscle strains and sprains are all disorders of this system and should be treated right at the onset.

■ DISORDERS OF THE MUSCULO-SKELETAL SYSTEM

The basic framework of our bodies is made up of bones. There are 208 bones in the body. These are placed together in such a manner as to give support, rigidity or stability; yet maintain balance, flexibility and mobility in different parts of the body, making us free to enjoy nature in all her beauty. This may be a walk in the garden, a swim in the lake, just lazing on the beach or to doing active exercises in the gym, swinging a golf club, sweeping the floor, cooking a meal—all physical activities essential to live life fully.

The junction between two bones is a joint. This approximation of the two bones to make a joint is facilitated by a band of fibrous tissue which attaches one bone to the other. These are called ligaments. The approximating body surfaces are covered by a tissue called cartilage. An encapsulated cushion with a certain amount of fluid and a soft yet firm membrane on the surface are called the articular capsule and the synovial membrane. The fluid secreted by this membrane is called the synovial fluid. To facilitate movement, there are bundles of tissue which are attached from one surface of the bone to another area. These are called muscles and the attaching ends are called tendons. To cushion movements, at the ends are small sac-like projections or bags of fluids called bursae. The actual joint site is called the articular surface. The general area of the joint, and that around it, not exactly right at the joint, are peri-articular surfaces. Those sites and structures involved in the movement, but not related to the bony joint, are extra-articular, for example, muscles, nerves, skin, tissue below the skin, and so forth.

ARTHRITIS

In a healthy state, all joint movements appear very smooth, fluid and easy, and one is actually unaware of them. They are taken for granted.

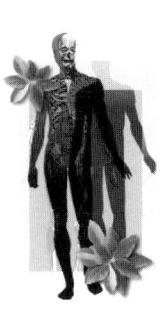

Causes and symptoms

However, movements at the joints are exposed to innumerable stresses in day-to-day life. These stresses expose them to stretches, strains, actual injury, or indirect injuries by infection due to various microbes. Metabolic disorders may deposit chemical crystals at the joint site, or immune system dysfunction may cause localised tissue lesions due to antigen, antibody reactions. This is not the end of the list. Degenerative changes in the body due to ageing, etc., take their own toll, e.g., osteo-arthritis. Cancerous growths at the site or nearby are another cause of dysfunction and disability. Dysfunction and disability are not due to a specific cause or disease entity. One specific cause may co-exist with another non-specific one, actually related to some other organ dysfunction.

Disease, dysfunction or disability of any of the areas mentioned above will cause pain, and maybe also swelling, disfigurement and loss of mobility.

Remedies

Herbal remedies have been found to be beneficial without the side effects of conventional drug therapy. These remedies, if not actually curative, are definitely complementary.

Before I begin to put down folk remedies for the treatment of arthritis, I must mention an observation I made during my stay at Barmer in Rajasthan. In this area, the water is high in flourides and one often comes across people who have been working / posted there complaining of joint pain. In this area, there is an abundant growth of the fenugreek plant, which is used extensively in culinary preparations. Its leaves are used to make a variety of dishes. Its seeds are not only used as a condiment, as elsewhere in India, but are also prepared as a main dish. A cupful of seeds are soaked overnight, the water drained the next day, and the seeds re-soaked in fresh water for a couple of hours. Then the water is changed a second time, and after a few hours, this

> ALL PAINS RELATED TO MUSCLE, BONE OR JOINT DISORDERS SHOULD BE INVESTIGATED AND TREATED SPECIFICALLY. HOWEVER, ARTHRITIS OR PAIN RELATED TO THESE STRUCTURES HAVE NO LASTING SOLUTIONS. IN MOST CASES, THERE IS ONLY PALLIATIVE CARE OR SLOWING THE PROGRESSION OF THE DISEASE PROCESS.

too is drained out. These seeds now are soft and tender, and are cooked as a dry vegetable or a curried pulse preparation. It is made at least 3-4 times a month. Apparently it prevents joint pain. The local population hardly ever complain of the type of joint pain the outsiders have. The people of this area are hardy, work on the land, and live off the land. They do not have joint pains/ deformity problems like those who come here to work for 2-3 years, and who do not have the same dietary habits as them. It seems that fenugreek seeds have some sort of substance that prevents fluoride salt deposits in the joint spaces.

■ Drinking beetroot juice or eating a cupful of diced beetroot, whether raw or parboiled, is extremely good for arthritis. The leaves of beetroot are also beneficial. These can be cooked with diced onions. Apparently, beetroots are supposed to have immunity-enhancing properties and are particularly beneficial for arthritis of an immune-disorder etiology. Beetroots are rich in potassium and have an alkalising effect. This alkalinity is helpful in dissolving various types of salt deposits on the articular surfaces of the joints, as occurs in arthritis. Those having beetroot may have pink-or red-coloured urine. This is because of the red pigment, fresh beta-cyanin, that some people do not metabolise well. However, this is no cause for worry.

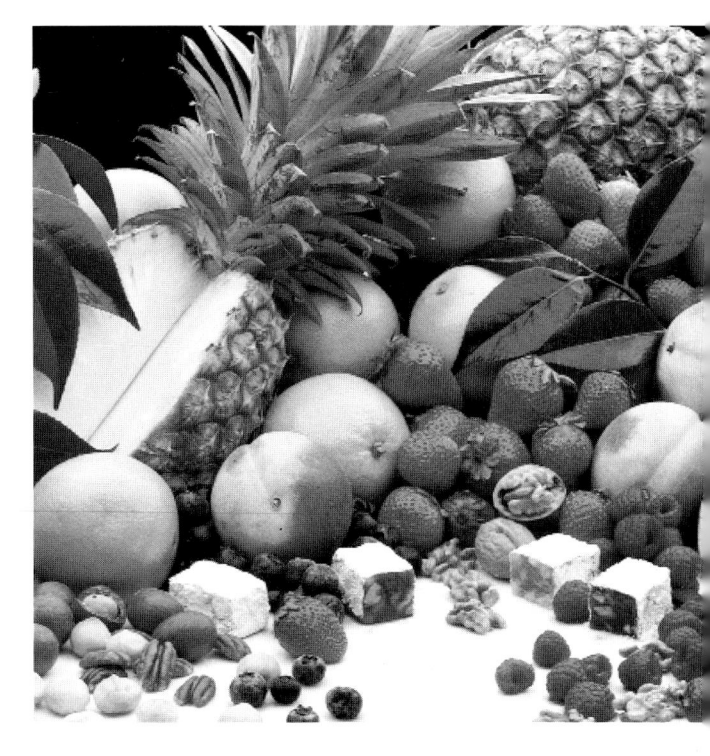

■ Pineapple juice, a cupful taken every day (200 ml), reduces swelling and inflammation around the joints, which occurs in rheumatoid arthritis and osteoarthritis. The active ingredient is a substance called bromelain that has significant anti- inflammatory action.

■ Apple-cider vinegar—vinegar made from apples: A tablespoonful taken with a teaspoon of honey in a glass of warm water first thing in the morning is

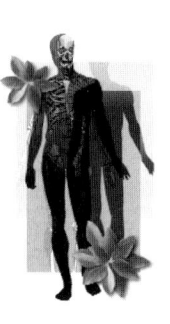

JUICES beneficial for treating arthritis are those obtained from carrots, spinach, celery, beet and cucumber. The effect of taking these juices, had separately, is far superior to that of a mixture. If a patient has the patience and will to try the juice therapy, three-fourth of a cup (150-200 ml) of each juice, freshly prepared, should be taken separately at an interval of three hours. This way the specific effect of each juice is felt, as just by symptoms it is not possible to ascertain what exactly is the inorganic salt combination deposited on the joint surfaces. Each type of arthritis has a different etiology. None of these juices are harmful. However, those with kidney stones will need to consult a physician before embarking on a sustained juice-treatment schedule. Spinach and tomatoes are harmful for those with kidney stones.

beneficial. Those who are not overweight can take more honey – a tablespoon or so. Apple-cider vinegar has a substance called mallic acid that helps remove inorganic salt deposits on articular surfaces—especially useful for non-specific arthritis.

■ Celery is another leafy vegetable used for salads or soup seasoning which has high amounts of sodium, which helps keep the balance of lime (calcium salt) and magnesium in solution, not letting it deposit on joint surfaces. The stalk and leaves can both be used to make fresh juice. By itself, this juice is not very palatable, so an equal amount of carrot juice can be added. A cupful of this mixture, taken morning and evening, prepared fresh and had immediately, will break down disease-producing unhealthy calcium deposits on the articular surfaces of joints. Cucumber juice can be substituted for celery juice once in a while.

■ Asparagus is good for those with arthritis, but definitely contraindicated for sufferers of gout. However, cherries are extremely good for relieving pain caused by gout.

■ Asparagus is beneficial, as well as its

seeds. Equal quantities of asparagus seeds, fenugreek seeds and black cummin seeds can be powdered and stored. One level teaspoon of this mixture taken every morning will relieve pain during the acute phase of the disease.

- Raw potato juice is beneficial for gout.

- The juice of bitter gourd is good for both gout and rheumatism.

- Wheatgrass or sprouted wheatgerm – half a cup taken daily—builds up the immune system and is especially good for all kinds of arthritis due to an autoimmune dysfunction, e.g., rheumatoid arthritis, systemic lupus erythromatosis and multiple sclerosis.

- Green gram is the new, fresh, just ready form of Bengal gram. Green gram is eaten in India as a green vegetable, like peas. The dried form is yellow or cream in colour. A soup made with a handful of green gram, boiled, mashed well and seasoned with 2-3 crushed cloves of garlic is a good seasonal remedy for pain in the joints—a cupful of soup twice a day. Some joint pains get aggravated in winter, and green gram is harvested only in the winter months. Nature provides us with timely cures, even though we are not aware of them.

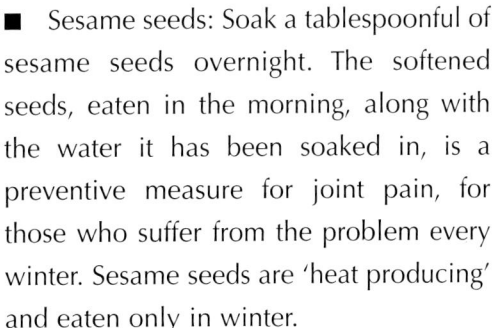

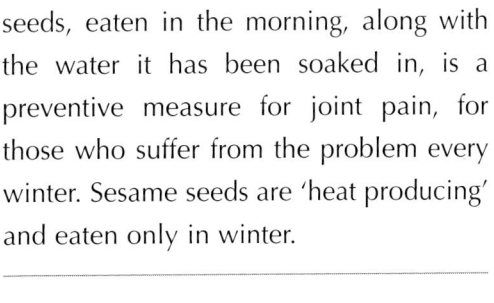

- Sesame seeds: Soak a tablespoonful of sesame seeds overnight. The softened seeds, eaten in the morning, along with the water it has been soaked in, is a preventive measure for joint pain, for those who suffer from the problem every winter. Sesame seeds are 'heat producing' and eaten only in winter.

- Fenugreek leaves, cooked in fresh coconut milk seasoned with garlic, has ingredients beneficial for seasonal joint-pain aggravation. It is a winter joint pain remedy.

- Chronic joint pains get relief after the patient has a herbal tea made from liquorice—a teaspoon of liquorice root stock in one cup of water. Boil for 5-6 minutes and drink it.

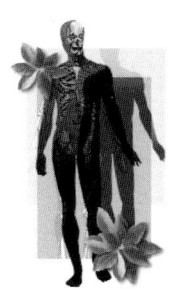

- Take equal quantities of dried ginger powder, cummin powder and add half the amount of black pepper powder. Grind together and store. Have half a teaspoon of this thrice a day. It has analgesic and anti-inflammatory properties. It is best to have this with water or fresh buttermilk that is not sour. By itself, it has a pungent taste, and may cause a little acidity for those with a pitta constitution.

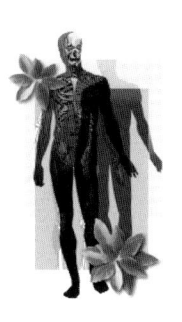

■ Chronic constipation or sluggish bowels are supposed to have a direct bearing on arthritis. Most ayurvedic remedies are first directed at this underlying condition. For those with joint pains, the classic remedy is the three-herb preparation, *triphala*—Indian gooseberry, *terminalia chebula* and *terminalia belerica*. A teaspoonful of this mixture, or even plain Indian gooseberry powder, taken with warm water at bedtime for a few days, regularises bowel movements. The high amount of vitamin-C in Indian gooseberry is extremely efficacious for all healing, repair, and wear and tear of tissues.

■ Half a teaspoon of castor oil in a cup of warm milk, taken 2-3 times a day, keeps the bowels clear. A pinch of powdered green cardamom, with sugar added to it, makes it palatable. Cardamom has a mildly constipating effect, but the combination of castor oil and cardamom naturally balances what the body needs to smoothen the passage of the contents of the bowel without any problem.

■ If you have castor growing near your house (it often grows wild, though it is usually cultivated in the fields), make a decoction using a 2"-piece of fresh or dried root. A tablespoon of this decoction taken twice a day gives relief to those with joint pain.

Causes and symptoms

■ Castor leaves warmed on a griddle

MASSAGES AND LOCAL APPLICATIONS

Swollen and painful joints need not only systemic oral medication, but locally applied soothing medicaments too. These applications must be bearably warm, bordering on hot but not so hot as to cause burns. They should not be kept on for more than 5-10 minutes. In some cases, there can be a local irritation. In that case, discontinue the treatment.

GARLIC

Botanical name: Allium sativum

Description and uses: The garlic plant is a member of the some group of plants as the onion. The bulb, the only part eaten or used, consists of numerous cloves grouped together and enclosed within a whitish skin. It is strong-smelling and pungent in taste, and is used in many parts of the world as a seasoning in food. The medicinal uses of garlic are legion. It is an antiseptic, a diuretic, an expectorant, a stimulant and a diaphoretic. Great healing powers have been ascribed to garlic, which is widely used to treat fever, hypertension, disorders of the nose, throat problems such as tonsillitis pharyngitis and laryngitis, chest pain, asthma, coughs, flatulence, diarrhoea, intestinal

smeared with warm castor oil, and placed on a painful joint, soothe the pain and relieves swelling. Just see that the leaves are warm and not burning hot. The idea is to give warmth, not to get burnt.

- A handful of pounded, mashed castor seeds, fried in a tablespoon of castor oil, placed in a muslin cloth and used as a poultice on the affected joint given relief.

- A similar preparation, made with a tablespoon of pounded mustard seeds, fried in mustard oil and made into poultice, is also effective.

- Onion juice, or warmed, mashed onion bulb, mixed with warm mustard oil, makes an effective poultice for arthritis.

- To 4-5 tender and green banyan leaves, add 4-5 cloves of garlic. Grind them to a paste and fry lightly in two tablespoons of sesame-seed oil. Cool slightly to a bearable temperature and add a tablespoon of kerosene oil to it. YES! kerosene oil. Mix well and apply this paste on the painful joints. Some villagers use kerosene oil only and swear by its efficacy.

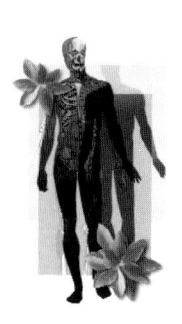

- The warm pulp of the aloe leaf soothes joint pains. It has an awful smell, hence some people prefer less smelly remedies!

- Body massage with warm neem oil 2-3 times a week is another remedy for rheumatoid pains.

- Take 2-4 tablespoons of mustard oil. Heat it. Fry 2-3 cloves of crushed garlic and a spoonful of pounded omum seeds in it. Cool it to a bearable temperature. Filter and use it to massage a painful joint.

- The fresh latex (milk) from the banyan twig, or the juice of the stems/leaves of the fig tree, applied on arthritic joints gives relief.

- Add a teaspoon of black pepper powder to a tablespoon of boiling hot sesame oil. Keep aside to cool a little. Filter and use while still warm as massage oil on painful rheumatoid joints.

SCIATICA / LUMBAGO

Pain in the lower back, radiating down to the legs on one or both sides, is referred to as sciatica. Low-back pain is a very common complaint in advancing years, though nowadays we hear the younger generation voicing similar sentiments.

Man belongs to the mammal family, and, like others mammals, was meant to walk on all four limbs. Somewhere up the evolution ladder he stood upright, and this posture subjected the lower spine to some amount of stress. Some adaptation of muscle development and movement minimised this, but the aging process brings about some inevitable degenerative changes coupled with the 'comforts' of sedentary, automated lifestyles, which makes sure that we do not exercise our muscles/ limbs to keep them in proper shape, tone and optimum functional capacity.

Causes and symptoms

There are various causes for low-back pain. These range from congenital factors, like a defect in the curvature of the spine, that makes weight-bearing not a healthy physiological function, but exerting stress on the spine, giving rise to a persistent backache.

Low backache could be a result of trauma, infection, growths, or referred pain from other sites.

Any injury to the backbone, i.e., individual vertebrae, puts stress / pressure on emerging nerve roots. If this pressure is too much, there may be paralysis of the areas the nerve root supplies. But just a wee bit of pressure, not enough to warrant active interference, gives rise to a persistent low backache. Sometimes, healing of soft-tissue injuries in the affected area can show excessive fibrosis and calcification in advancing years, resulting in old injury areas becoming painful in advancing years.

Fractures of the cartilaginous disc between two vertebrae, or its prolapse into the vertebrae canal, puts pressure on the spinal cord, causing backache. Degenerative processes can also cause a similar problem.

Infections of internal organs, muscles, nerves in any specific area next to the spine, will also cause pressure symptoms/pain, e.g., tuberculosis or shingles.

There are causes other than infection which can produce inflammatory changes in the vertebral joints, resulting in stiffness, rigidity and pain, particularly after a period of rest, e.g., ankylosing spondylitis or bamboo spine. Aging causes general wear and tear of the cartilage around the joints, leading to degenerative changes, and some bony outgrowths take place, pressing on nerve roots, e.g. osteoarthritis and osteophytes.

In metabolic disorders like osteoporosis, osteomalasia or chondrocalcinosis, the calcium laying down and removal from bony tissue is deranged. Herpes zoster, a viral infection of the nerve root, secondary cancers, etc., may all be causes of low backache.

A physiological cause of low backache is pregnancy, wherein the abdominal and back muscles are stretched. Similar stresses occur in obesity or pelvic and abdominal disorders.

The causes enumerated above are to emphasise that a persistent low backache should not be neglected but examined by an orthopaedician, if home remedies do not help. These, at best, are palliative or complementary, and real treatment may be more specific, whether it is treatment by drugs, surgery or orthopaedic manipulation.

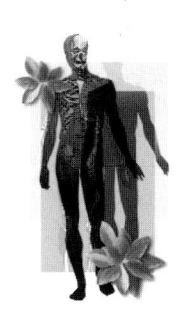

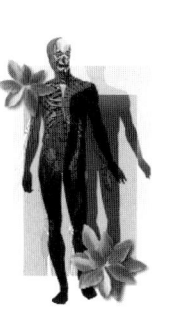

BACKACHE

A pain referred along the distribution of the sciatic nerve, which supplies the lower limbs, is referred to as sciatica. Any backache which is the result of mechanical stretches, strains, ligamentous tears, or a ruptured intervertebral disc, is very sudden and severe. Pains that are related to pelvic or abdominal organ dysfunction might not be that severe, barring kidney pain, e.g., renal colic or pain due to stones anywhere in the urinary tract.

Remedies

The remedies suggested below are for non-specific backache—backache where a cause has not been found and is attributed to arthritis or aging. No manipulation or massage should be done unless an X-ray rules out the presence of a prolapsed intervertebral disc, dislocation or fracture.

Note: *All remedies suggested for arthritis will help to alleviate pain.*

Eat all food that is high in vitamin-C. Cabbage, guava, kiwi, papaya and the poor man's all-purpose fruit, Indian gooseberry, the highest source of natural vitamin-C. This is retained even when the fruit is cooked. Just having one fourth of a dried Indian gooseberry will suffice.

There are specific yogic exercises for relieving back pain. Consult a yoga teacher for expert advice.

MUSCLE SPRAINS/STRAINS/TENDONITIS

Muscles are specialised cells and tissues which are placed together as a bundle or organ, which by its contraction produces movement in an organism. The ends of each muscle organ have specialised cells which are strong and fibrous, yet maintain the elasticity of the muscles. These cells form attachments to bones or cartilage, to form an anchorage from where the action of movement begins or ends. These ends are called tendons. Similar cell and tissue collections are present between the bony ends of the participating bones of a joint, which support and strengthen movement in a joint. These are called ligaments and are attached either to the bony ends of joints or the cartilage covering them.

Causes and symptoms

When strenuous exercise is done without adequate warming up, or sudden movement takes place at a joint, these muscle or ligament fibres get over-stretched and even torn, resulting in a strain. When fibres of the cartilaginous capsule covering a joint get torn, it is called a sprain. When there is displacement of bony surfaces from their normal position during such an injury, it results in a dislocation. The shoulder, elbow, knee and ankle joint are very susceptible to sudden stresses. Such injuries usually result in swelling at the site. A swelling, which slowly develops at the site of the muscle/tendon injury, is usually a sprain. This is due to bleeding within the joint cavity. It takes 24-48 hours for a sprain to show up with a swelling. In sprains, some movement, though painful, is still possible, but in a dislocation or fracture there is no movement possible, and obvious deformity will be immediately visible.

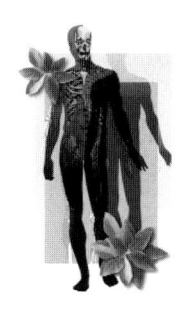

Remedies

■ Take two tablespoons of sesame-seed or sunflower oil (or any cooking medium), add a tablespoon of turpentine or kerosene to it, and then apply it as a linament.

■ Half a teaspoonful of camphor, added to one-fourth cup of sunflower oil and gently massaged/ rubbed in, soothes a sprain.

■ A few cloves of garlic, pounded and mixed with olive or mustard oil, applied with a warm bandage/poultice, gives relief from pain.

ALWAYS REST A SUSPECTED SPRAIN/STRAIN. A COLD COMPRESS OR CRUSHED ICE SHOULD BE PLACED ON THE PAINFUL AREA IMMEDIATELY. IT PREVENTS A SWELLING. NEXT APPLY A PRESSURE BANDAGE—NOT TIGHT, JUST COMFORTABLE—AND PLACE THE LIMB IN AN ELEVATED POSITION. ONCE SWELLING HAS OCCURRED, BATHING A SPRAIN WITH WARM WATER TO WHICH SALT HAS BEEN ADDED BRINGS RELIEF.

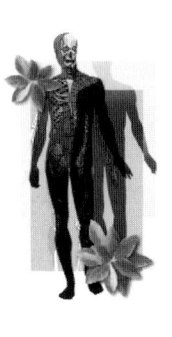

- A teaspoon of fresh ginger paste, to which a level teaspoon of turmeric powder is added, should be applied liberally on the sprain area and bandaged lightly. If there is a swelling already, then add a little salt to this paste.

- Crush a handful of eucalyptus leaves, a few cloves, 10-12 mint leaves, a few sprigs of coriander leaves, and grind them together. Add 1-2 tablespoons of very warm coconut oil, and apply locally. This will give temporary relief while its warm.

Note: *Any of the massage oils/poultices for arthritis can be applied locally. All these relieve pain. However, even if it is rested, the sprain will still take 5-7 days to get better.*

MUSCLE CRAMPS

Painful muscular contractions are called cramps. They can occur at any time and can be very painful and uncomfortable.

Causes and symptoms

These usually occur in the leg muscles after a particular heavy bout of unscheduled, strenuous muscular activity / exercise, when a person has perspired a lot and the weather is very warm. Intense cold can also cause cramps. Continuous use of a certain group of muscles, as in writing, can cause cramps in the fingers / hand.

Remedies

- Gentle massaging of the area which has cramps gives relief. Maintain adequate hydration levels. After exercise, drink water to which salt and sugar have both been added. Some women get cramps in their legs during pregnancy. This only needs gentle massage to get rid of the problem.

Note: *Frozen shoulder, housemaids's knee, clergyman's knee, tennis elbow, are names given to pain in these areas, due to either a local stress injury, which has not been rested, or an overuse injury. All remedies to relieve pain—gentle massage, exercise under supervision, physiotherapy, are recommended.*

ASPARAGUS

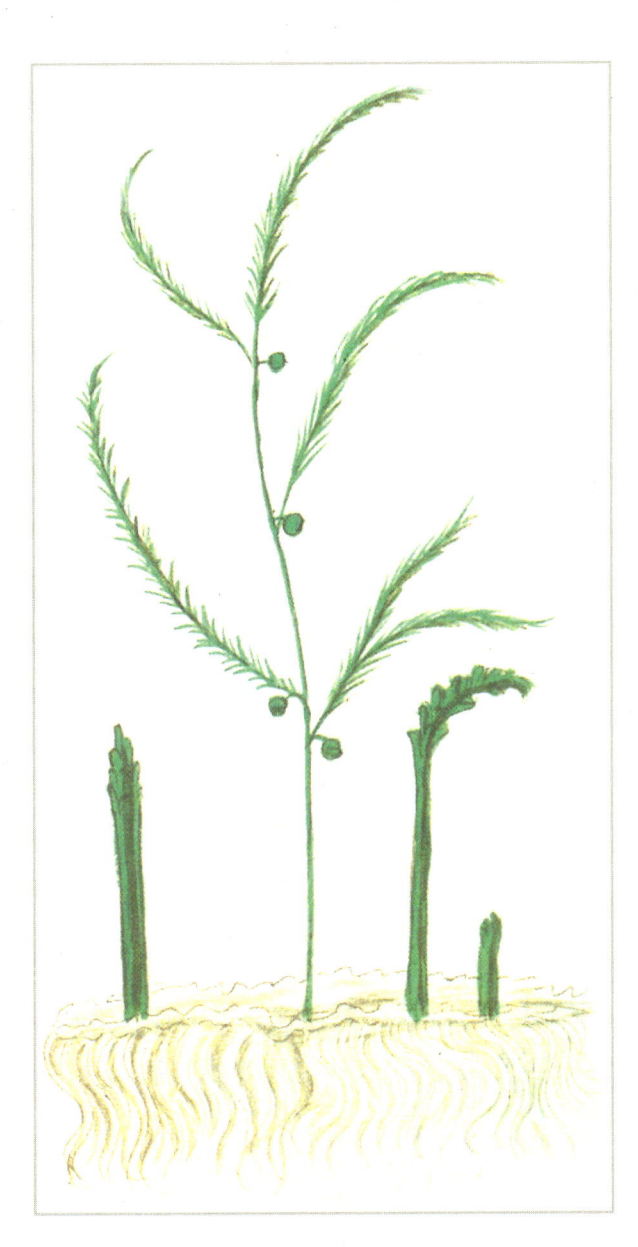

Botanical name:
Asparagus afficinalis

Description and uses: Asparagus is a popular table delicacy in the West. The young shoots and leaves are edible. Apart from its value as a food, asparagus is well known as a diuretic and a laxative. It has been found beneficial in cases of oedema, and used to treat general weakness and debility, arthritis, sexual debility and excessive menstruation. Asparagus is also known to improve eyesight, soothe a toothache and augment lactation in nursing mothers.

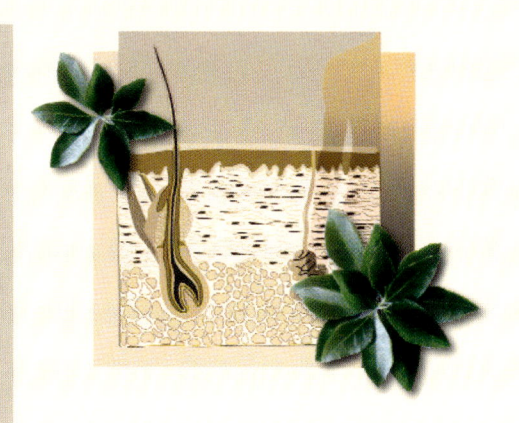

Our bodies are covered entirely by our skin, which not only protects us from the external elements, but also makes us aware of touch, pain, heat and cold. It is delicate and prone to numerous problems. Therefore, preventing or successfully treating skin disorders is of paramount importance.

SKIN PROBLEMS

Our entire body is encapsulated in a protective covering—the skin. It has the unique capacity to adapt and protect us from hot and cold weather, the sun, the wind, and the numerous organisms in the atmosphere. The skin has two layers—an outer layer, the epidermis, and an inner layer, the dermis. Underneath, and in these layers, are present a network of fine nerve endings and blood vessels. The skin makes us aware of touch, pain and temperature. It has numerous pores, which are openings of sweat glands situated in the dermis. These glands are organs of excretion. They excrete excess salts, help maintain the salt and water balance of the body, and complement other organs of excretion, principally the kidneys and bowels, and to some extent the lungs.

The skin, besides being exposed to the elements—air, wind, rain, sun, etc.—is also extremely sensitive to infections and environmental pollutants. To remain healthy, it is important to keep it healthy and clean. Personal cleanliness is very important. It includes daily, regular bathing, and using oils or creams to keep the surface of the skin smooth and soft. Despite all the care taken, some problems still arise, which need a little more consideration than just a regular bath and good hygiene.

The concept of starting out with a baby-soft skin at birth is wonderful, but some infants are covered with a white, waxy substance all over their bodies, more so in the crevices—in the armpits, groin, elbows, behind the knees, and also on the scalp. This is called cradle cap or *vernix caseosa*. Some babies have it only on the scalp. However, it is not a serious problem—it is a natural protective substance which keeps the foetal skin healthy when it remains in a watery environment for nine months. *Vernix caseosa* comes off gradually on its own by the end of six weeks—which is the normal postnatal period needed for the mother to recuperate. At birth, the attendant normally wipes some of it off gently with a soft, damp, clean cloth. The baby is bathed in some hospitals, but some patients who have had domicillary deliveries, prefer not to bathe the baby till the cord dries completely and falls off—usually in 7-8 days.

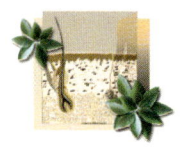

Remedies

■ Those of you who would like to bath your baby daily, if the weather is warm enough, could use olive oil or sesame-seed oil to gently massage the baby. A swab soaked in oil can be gently rubbed in the armpits, behind the knees, and on the scalp. It takes off the excess waxy substance. Then bathe the baby with warm water, using a mild soap. Remember to dry the scalp and body well. But do not rub the baby's skin. If you are too vigorous in your cleaning schedule, the soft skin will get damaged, abraised and infected. So take care. In time, this substance will disappear.

NAPPY RASH

The advent of modern conveniences has bought its share of side effects. The practice of using disposable nappies / diapers with a plastic shield has given rise to many more cases of nappy rash, as compared to earlier days.

Causes and symptoms

Nappy rash occurs in the region of the groin in babies because this area is often not cleaned properly and kept dry. The old practice of keeping a baby's bottom bare, or using soft cotton nappies, was good, even though it meant frequent changing of the baby's bedsheet and a lot of additional washing for the mother. There are certain solutes and bacteria in baby urine which per se cause no problem, but prolonged contact with the skin, and dampness in the area, gives rise to rough, raw-looking, angry red skin, which may get infected and cause a weeping eczema-like condition. This may be localised in the genital area or spread to the thighs, buttocks, etc. Detergents used to wash nappies, using harsh soaps or bleaches to clean them, inadequate rinsing in clean, clear water, or improper drying, can also cause a rash. Sometimes the mother's diet may have some ingredients that are passed out in her milk, which do not agree with the baby. Some babies may have a milk-allergy rash. The rash is then not limited to the nappy area.

Remedies

■ Eliminate the commonest cause for the rash. Use dry nappies which have

OLIVE

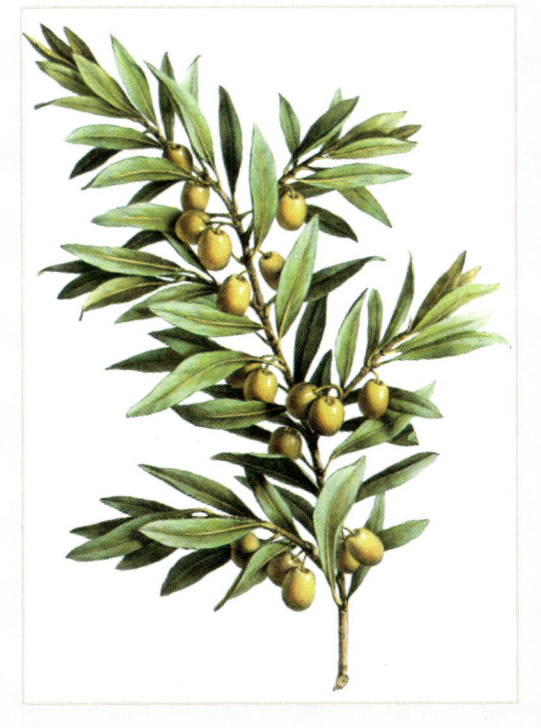

Botanical name: *Olea Europaea*

Description and uses: The olive tree, an evergreen of the genus *olea*, and it has dark green, lance-shaped leathery leaves which have silvery undersides. Olive is a small, oval fruit with a hard stone and bitter flesh—green when unripe, and bluish black when ripe. The fleshy part of the fruit is filled with oil. This oil is extracted and used for innumerable purposes.

Olive oil is a demulcent and laxative; it relieves pruritis, stings and burns, and is a good vehicle for liniments. As a lubricant, it is valuable for skin, muscular, joint, kidney and chest complaints. It is also highly efficacious in the treatment of problems related to the head and ears, nappy rash in babies, corns, calluses, morning sickness in pregnancy, and stretch marks on the skin.

been washed with a non-toxic detergent or soap, and then rinsed well in several changes of clean water. Keep the groin area dry

■ A light application of coconut oil or olive oil on the affected area is soothing for a rash. It acts as a barrier cream.

■ Wash the baby's bottom with water in which neem leaves have been boiled—a handful of neem leaves in 2-3 litres of water. Leave the leaves in the water till it cools. Filter and use this water.

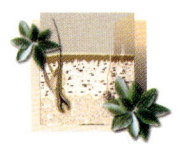

RASHES DUE TO MEASLES, CHICKEN POX, HEAT RASH, PRICKLY HEAT

One breaks into a rash in measles, chicken pox, heat rash or prickly heat. This takes its course, and although the discomfort can be soothed and alleviated somewhat, the rash will not go away immediately.

Remedies

- Apply a thin layer of sandalwood paste on the rash-affected areas.

- If there are any pustules or lesions, a paste of sandalwood with neem leaves can be applied. A teaspoon of sandalwood powder mixed with half a teaspoon of neem powder, with a little rose water to moisten it, made into a paste, should be applied to the effected area.

- Fresh coriander-leaf paste is also soothing for heat rashes.

- For measles, bath the area with warm water to which a tablespoon of apple-cider vinegar has been added, or water in which green peas have been boiled. Strain and use the water.

SUNBURN

The sun gives warmth and is very welcome on a cold wintry day. However, it rays can also cause sunburn when the skin is exposed to strong sunlight for long hours, as some people find out to their discomfort.

Causes and symptoms

Sunburn is a result of deleterious ultra-violet rays, which in small measures gives a lovely tan, but in larger doses can cause blistering.

Sunburn affects young and fair skin more than dark skin. It causes early aging of the skin, which loses its elasticity.

Remedies

- Bath the sunburnt area with water to which bakin soda has been added. A tablespoonful to a bucket of water will suffice.

- Add a tablespoon of apple-cider

vinegar to a bucketful of water for bathing.

- Cucumber slices or grated cucumber placed in a damp cloth, and chilled, and used as a cold compress on the sunburnt area, is very soothing.

- Aloe vera: Fresh leaf juice or pulp applied to the sunburnt area/blisters will heal the skin surface painlessly.

- An infusion of marigold flowers can be used as a face wash.

SANDALWOOD

Botanical name: *Santalum album*

Description and uses: Sandalwood is the scented wood of a tree of the genus *santalum—in* full white sandalwood. A yellow aromatic oil is extracted from it.

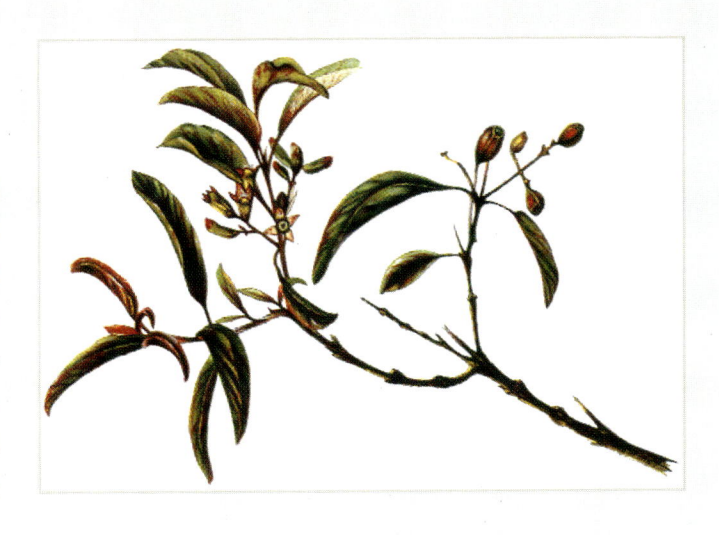

Sandalwood oil, paste and powder are the panacea for a host of ailments. The oil promotes mental balance, a feeling of peace and tranquility, and a cool, relaxed mind. The paste and powder are used for hypertension; the paste for headache, rashes caused by measles, chicken pox, heat rash, prickly heat, acne, allergic rash and eczema; and the powder for white patches on the skin.

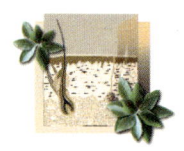

BLISTERS

A blister is a collection of fluid in a pocket of the outer layer of the skin.

Causes and symptoms

Infection, friction, sunburn, burns, viral infection like chicken pox, all cause blisters. Other causes are skin problems such as eczema, frictional damage caused by ill-fitting shoes, long walking trips, treks, and so forth. Blisters can be very painful, especially if they burst and the raw skin is exposed.

Remedies

- Skin a fresh aloe leaf and apply the pulp or juice on the blister.

- Crush a clove of garlic. To a drop of its juice, add a drop of olive oil, and apply it on the blister.

- Fresh spring onion juice can also be locally applied.

A BLISTER HEALS BEST ON ITS OWN. DO NOT ATTEMPT TO BURST A BLISTER UNLESS IT IS IN AN AREA WHERE IT IS CAUSING PAIN DUE TO PRESSURE, OR IS LIKELY TO BURST DUE TO UNAVOIDABLE FRICTION WITH CLOTHES, ETC. IN THAT CASE PUNCTURE IT. USE A NEEDLE WHICH HAS BEEN STERILISED BY HOLDING IT OVER A FLAME—DO NOT LET THE SOOT COLLECT ON IT, AND HOLD THE POINT IN THE BLUE PART OF THE FLAME. WHEN THE POINT BECOMES RED HOT, REMOVE IT FROM THE FLAME AND WAVE IT IN THE AIR TO COOL IT. THE NEEDLE CAN ALSO BE STERILISED BY PLACING IT IN ALCOHOL. ONCE PUNCTURED, THE FLUID WILL DRAIN OUT FROM THE BLISTER. DO NOT TRY REMOVING THE REST OF THE SKIN. COVER WITH A CLEAN DRESSING DURING THE DAY AND LEAVE IT UNCOVERED AT NIGHT, TO LET IT DRY.

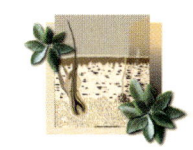

CHILBLAINS

Chilblains are the unprotected skin's response to extreme cold. The lesions caused are on the extremities, the toes and fingers.

Causes and symtpoms

In chilblains, freezing causes the terminal blood vessels to shut down. This is called vasoconstriction. The local tissue metabolism being at an extremely low ebb, the requirement for oxygen is much more, due to the extreme cold. Vasoconstriction decreases blood supply, which leads to tissue damage. Chilblains are itchy, red skin lesions, with or without a slight swelling, or even blistering, at the site. The swelling increases when heat is applied to give warmth. Untreated, or unheeded, these become haemorrhagic and even infected. Prevention, in this, as in most cases, is better than cure. Keep warm, be adequately clothed, keep dry and keep moving. Avoid smoking.

Remedies

- The part of the body that has chilblains should be elevated. This will reduce the swelling. Stay indoors in a warm room and let the body adjust to the warm room temperature naturally. Only then start with gentle, slow massage.

- Grind a few black peppercorns and fry them in a tablespoonful of hot mustard or sesame-seed oil. Filter, and while still warm, use this oil for massage. Make sure the skin is not abraded or bruised, or else this will cause pain and inflammation.

- A folk remedy is to make a paste with a tablespoonful of honey, glycerine, egg white and wholemeal flour. Spread this over the chilblain and leave it overnight. This forms an insulation from the cold and lets the body heal from within. Wash it off with warm water in the morning.

- Regular massage of hands and feet in winter with any warmed vegetable oil, with a few drops of lemon added, improves circulation. Use the discarded halves of lemons to cup them around fingers/toes, and rub them for a while. Wash off with warm water.

- Soak hands/feet in a warm infusion of marigold flowers to which a spoonful of sea salt has been added.

- Fresh onion juice, or a poultice made

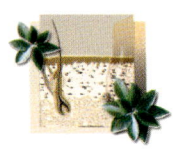

of leeks/spring onions, placed while warm (not hot) on areas prone to chilblains, acts as a preventive and also has curative value.

■ Similarly, fresh garlic juice and warm oil also helps in reducing itching. Rinse out hands in warm water, or the pungent garlic smell will remain.

■ A poultice of hot potato paste, with a few drops of glycerine, applied every night to fingers and toes prone to chilblains, is a preventive and cure for painful swelling.

■ Warm broken wheat or oatmeal porridge can also be used to dip the fingers in, as a cure for chilblains.

CHAPPED LIPS AND DRY SKIN

Chapped lips and dry skin are a problem people have a contend with in dry climates. They need constant care and attention.

Causes and symptoms

Winter days and cold winds are especially harsh to the skin. There is low humidity and the skin becomes dry and the lips chapped. The skin is exposed to cold winds and gets depleted of natural oils. Washing hands repeatedly with detergents and soaps also takes its toll.

Remedies

■ A body massage with any vegetable oil, followed by a warm-water bath in winter, smoothens dry skin.

■ An oatmeal or gram-flour face pack, to which fresh yoghurt and cream and a pinch of turmeric is added, helps clear the face of dry skin. This can also be used to bathe with, as a substitute for soap.

■ A face pack of powdered lentils, fresh cream and turmeric works the same way. The lentils should be soaked overnight

APPLY A LITTLE GHEE OR BUTTER IN THE UMBLICUS (BELLY BUTTON) AT BEDTIME. THIS IS A FOLK REMEDY THAT HEALS DRY, CHAPPED LIPS. HOW THIS ACTS IS DEBATABLE, BUT ACT IT DOES!

MARIGOLD

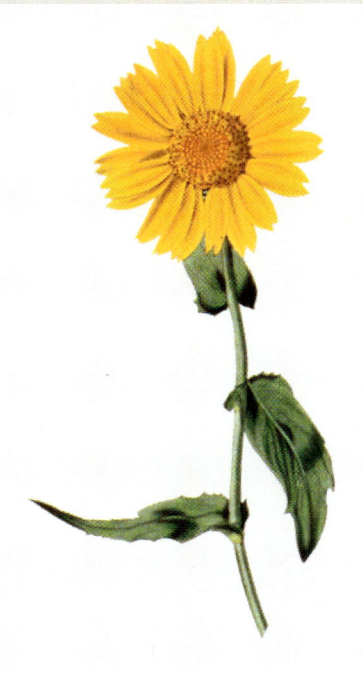

Botanical name: *Calendula officinalis*

Description and uses: The marigold is a familiar flower, with its pale-green leaves and golden or golden-orange petals. This easily available flower is used to prepare herbal remedies for problems related to the head, sunburn, chilblains, body adour, herpes, psoriasis, stress-related disorders, scanty periods, chronic ulcers and varicose veins. Internal administration assists local action and suppuration. It is, however, generally used externally as a local application.

and then ground to a paste. Some people are allergic to gram flour, so lentils are a good substitute.

■ Equal portions of glycerine, rose water and fresh lime juice, mixed together and stored in a bottle, can be kept on the bathroom shelf. In winter, apply this all over the body after a hot-water bath. Leave it on for a minute and then pat the skin dry with a good absorbant towel. The towel takes away the stickiness of glycerine and leaves a warm, clean feeling all over the body.

WHITLOW

Infection of the nail bed is called whitlow. All the remedies given for boils are applicable for whitlow.

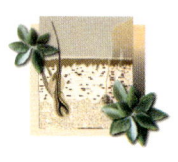

BOILS/FURUNCLE/CARBUNCLE

A boil is a localised hair-follicular infection. Each hair root has a bulbous base, and if it gets infected, a boil erupts.

Causes and symtoms

A run-down physical condition, neglect of personal hygiene, the accidental pulling out of a hair root, all are an invitation to microbes. These microbes are present on the skin all the time, and under normal, healthy, clean conditions cause no harm, but if and when they do get a chance, they infect the hair base, and a boil erupts. A boil is usually a localised, tender, pus-filled area surrounded by an angry, red circumscribed periphery. Incipient boils are red, raised swellings. They ripen slowly, and after that a pus-point forms in the centre. During this initial starting and ripening phase, there may be fever, malaise and extreme pain at the site. The boil comes to a head with a pus-point forming, which soon bursts. Once a boil bursts, the pain lessens and healing starts from the base, leaving a scar when healed. A deep-seated infection of the entire length of the hair follicle is called a furuncle. Furuncles may coalase together to form an abscess. Diabetes mellitus predisposes to boils. These boils do not heal easily and are called carbuncles.

Note: *Never try to break open a boil with a pin or a needle. And do not neglect one, especially if it is on the head and neck area. The blood circulation in these areas is such that infection can easily travel from there to the brain—with fatal results.*

Remedies

■ First wash and clean the area with soap water or a neem decoction.

■ Neem heads the list in herbal cures for boils. Grind fresh, tender leaves to a fine paste and apply daily on the boil.

■ Soak overnight 2-3 ripe pods of the neem fruit in a cup of water. Next morning, mash the pulp, add a little honey and drink this mixture. This cleanses the system from within.

■ Half a teaspoon of dried neem-leaf powder, taken once a day with a glass of hot water for 5-7 days is also a good internal cleanser. To make it palatable, add a teaspoon of honey to it.

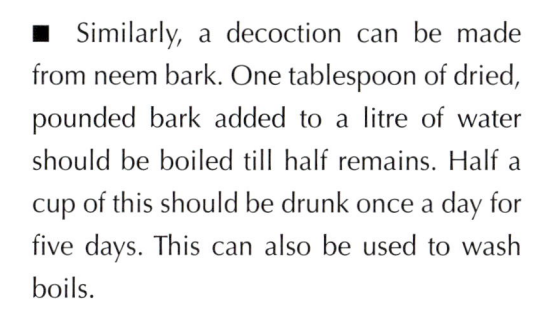

- Similarly, a decoction can be made from neem bark. One tablespoon of dried, pounded bark added to a litre of water should be boiled till half remains. Half a cup of this should be drunk once a day for five days. This can also be used to wash boils.

- Mash 2-3 fresh garlic cloves into a paste and apply locally on the boil.

- To bring a boil to head, roast a medium-sized onion over a fire. Mash. Make a poultice and apply over the boil while still warm. You can add a teaspoon of turmeric powder and a little hot ghee to this. Apply this poultice 2-3 times a day.

- Use oatmeal or wholegrain wheat flour to make a poultice. Fry a tablespoonful of flour in 1-2 teaspoons of coconut oil. Place on a muslin cloth and apply on the boil while still warm. Do this 3-4 times a day. The boil will come to a head and burst.

- Banyan/ castor / betel leaves—any of these, warmed with a little warm castor oil applied on the smooth surface, placed on the boil and bandaged, brings the boil to a head.

- A roasted, fresh fig leaf, cut in half and applied on the boil, makes a good poultice.

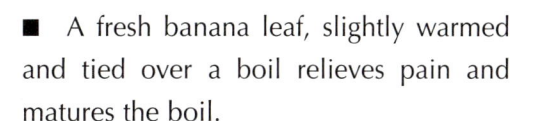

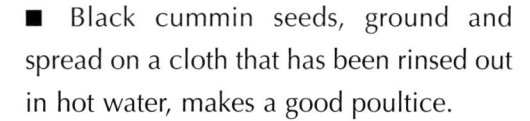

- A fresh banana leaf, slightly warmed and tied over a boil relieves pain and matures the boil.

- Black cummin seeds, ground and spread on a cloth that has been rinsed out in hot water, makes a good poultice.

- Finely ground pomegranate rind, mixed with a little hot mustard oil to make a paste, makes a fine poultice.

- Fenugreek seeds boiled in water, coarsely pounded, can be applied on a boil as a poultice.

- Turmeric paste: Use equal parts of fresh ginger and turmeric ground together. Apply when quite warm on a boil.

- Aloe pulp heals boils. Either the leaves can be washed and crushed to a paste, or the pulp can be extracted and used as a daily dressing for 3-5 days.

- When a boil just begins, if fresh henna-leaf paste is applied, it aborts the boil.

- Flowers of the flame of the forest tree:

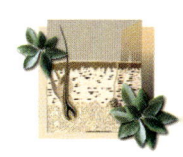

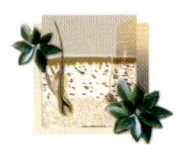

Take one or two flowers, steam and mash them, apply it on a boil and bandage it. It heals boils and even ulcers.

■ Take a tender colocasia leaf, crush and burn it to an ash. Mix a little hot sesame-seed oil to make a paste. Apply on boil the and bandage it. The leaves have an astringent and styptic action.

■ Bark of the peepul tree: To a tablespoonful of bark, ground to a fine paste, add hot milk or hot ghee. Apply on the boil as a poultice.

■ Cut a carrot into large pieces. Boil and mash it. Add a teaspoon of hot mustard oil to it and use it as a poultice.

■ Soak a slice of bread in hot water, to which a spoonful of mustard powder is added. Place this on a fine muslin cloth and use as a poultice while still very warm.

■ Those who have a tendency to repeated crops of boils should drink one-fourth of a cup of fresh bitter-gourd juice daily for a week. They should also get their blood sugar checked to eliminate the possibility of diabetes.

ABSCESS

An abscess can be extremely troublesome and cause great distress. It often takes very long to heal.

Causes and symptoms

When there is infection and disintegration of localised tissue, a cavity forms with a collection of pus. This too ripens like a boil, bursts and drains out. This is an abscess. An abscess needs to be drained out by surgical intervention.

Remedies

■ Once an abscess has been drained, it can be dressed with neem-leaf paste or garlic and turmeric paste.

■ Aloe pulp also heals a drained abscess site.

HENNA

Botanical name:
Lawsonia inermis

Description and uses:
Henna is a tropical shrub, 8- to 10- feet high, with small pink, red or white, sweet-smelling flowers.

Henna-leaf paste is used in India to decorate women's hands and feet—the intricate designs made with the paste are kept on for a while, and them washed off, leaving behind beautiful brownish-orange patterns. It is also popular as a hair conditioner and colourant.

Henna leaves have an astringent action and antibacterial properties. For pains, a paste made of the leaves, applied on the affected area, is soothing and gives relief. Gargling with an infusion made of henna leaves heals a sore throat; and burns, skin infections, jaundice, leprosy, smallpox are cured by using henna internally and locally. The juice of the leaf helps greatly in relieving vaginal discharge.

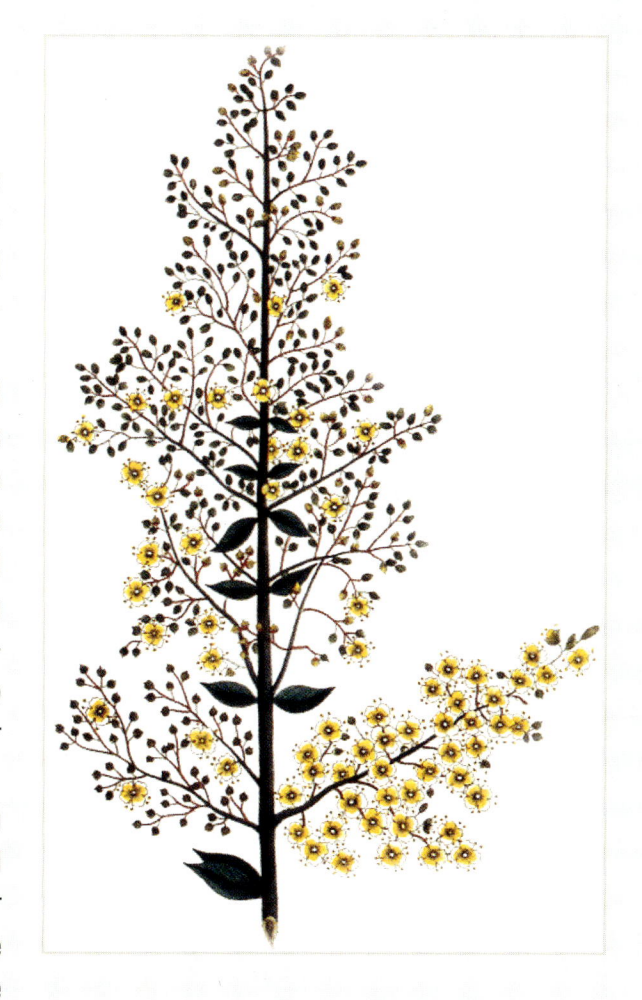

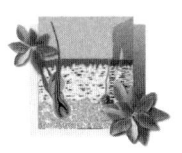

SCABIES

Scabies is a parasitic infection of the skin caused by a transmissible parasite, a mite—the female sarcoptis scabei.

Causes and symptoms

This parasite burrows into the superficial layer of skin, especially in the crevices of the body. It lays eggs, and the larvae hatch within a few days and surround the base of a hair follicle as it emerges from the skin. The body reacts to this parasite by causing a localised hypersensitivity reaction, which then results in intense itching, causing further spread and secondary superimposed infection by other microbes. This itching is marked during the night, and the eggs fall off on bedclothes / linen and spread to other people in the family. The itching is so severe that sometimes the skin looks raw. This infection can be identified by fine waxy lines or burrows on the sides of the fingers, in the webs of the fingers/toes, inner sides of the wrists, elbows, armpits, knees, groin area and the areola of the breast. Once secondary infection occurs, it is more difficult to pinpoint it as scabies.

Remedies

■ The best remedy for scabies is neem-leaf paste made with fresh or dried neem leaves and an equal quantity of turmeric powder mixed with mustard oil. This should be applied on the body and left for an hour or so. Then the person should bathe. Repeat for 7-10 days till all lesions have healed. The clothes should be washed and rinsed out after they have been soaked in boiled neem water. Simultaneously, the patient should be made to drink a tablespoon of neem-leaf or neem-bark decoction. Mustard oil may be an irritant for some skins, so do not leave it on for very long.

■ Neem-leaf paste can be made with only turmeic too, with no mustard oil. In this case, the patient should have a bath, apply the paste everywhere on the body, in-between the fingers, webs of toes, etc., and let it dry. Then he should put on clean clothes. Next day, he should not bathe. Fresh paste should be applied again. This should be done for three days. On the fourth day, the patient should have a warm-water bath and wear fresh clothes.

■ The dried bark of a peepul tree can be powdered fine, strained through a fine sieve, and used as a dusting powder on scabiotic lesions.

■ Extract the juice from 400-500 gm of drumstick leaves. Mix with an equal amount of sesame-seed oil, and boil till the water dries up. Cool and store. Apply daily over the infected parts. Both have a strong anti-microbial action, and sesame-seed oil is also insecticidal.

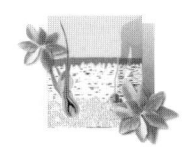

FUNGAL INFECTIONS

Ringworm, athlete's foot, jock itch, barber's itch, and tinea infection of the scalp and nails—in common language, all fungal infections of the skin are referred to as 'ringworm' infection.

Causes and function

Fungal infections thrive on dead necrotic tissue. Skin, hair, nails, scalp are actually dead tissue, the cornified layer of the skin. When this layer is scratched, the fungal organism gets access to underlying layers and causes a lesion. Fungal spores are present everywhere in the atmosphere, and also reside on the skin. In a debilitated physical health, or when there is poor personal hygiene, these spores take root and cause a localised, mild inflammation—there is only a slight redness to identify it. It gets further neglected and slowly spreads, giving rise to circumscribed lesions like a ring. The central areas heal and clear, while the peripheral areas keep getting spaced out and spread out. In some cases, an allergic reaction occurs. There is much itching and bullae formation. Otherwise, except for its appearance and spread it does not bother the patient much. Depending on the site, it is called athlete's foot, jock itch, barber's itch, and tinea infection on the scalp or nails. When these lesions appear on the body, they appear as annular lesions. In-between the toes, they are macerated white patches with scaly borders. They cause the nails to thicken, lose lustre, and the debris of tissue destruction get imbedded under the edges. In the jock area, a ringed lesion appears on the inner side of the thigh, which itches a lot, causing discomfort. This too is primarily caused by wearing tight-fitting synthetic garments which do not 'breath', and predispose to fungal and secondary infection. On the chin and beard area, they appear as small boils. On the scalp, they are ring-shaped and cause lustreless bald patches with small scales and sparse dull hair, finally causing a large bald patch. All bald pates are not a result of fungal infection!

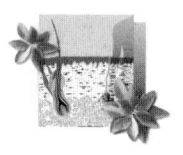

Fungal infection spreads slowly, insidiously, hence gets neglected in the initial phases.

Remedies

Of paramount importance is good personal hygiene, daily bathing and no sharing of personal garments, regular shampooing of the scalp, and drying the skin properly. Cotton or woollen clothes are more body-friendly than synthetics.

■ Grind a tablespoon of black gram to a paste with water. Add half a teaspoon of honey so that the mixture is of a mildly sticky consistency. Apply on the fungal patches in a thin layer.

■ Grind tamarind seeds and add fresh lime juice to make a paste. Apply daily for a few days.

■ Make a paste with fresh henna leaves. Take a tablespoonful, add a teaspoon each of turmeric powder and sesame-seed oil. Apply daily. This is especially good for athlete's foot.

■ If raw turmeric is available, grind and apply its juice.

■ The juice of fresh holy basil leaves or leaf paste is equally efficacious.

■ Mustard-seed paste also gives good results but it may irritate some skins, so check for a reaction.

■ Flame of the forest seeds: Apply the paste, made with a teaspoon of the seeds and a teaspoon of fresh lime juice, on the affected area. The seeds can also be dried, powdered and used as a dusting powder on the lesions—especially for those with an obstinate, recurrent infection.

■ Cluster beans: The leaves of this plant make an ideal medicated paste. Take a teaspon of the paste and a teaspoon each of fresh lime juice and fresh ginger paste. Mix together and apply.

■ Apply locally the bark of the root of the drumstick plant, made into a paste with water. The bark can also be dried, powdered and stored.

■ Use water for bathing in which a handful of neem leaves have been boiled.

- Fresh mint juice can also be applied on the infected skin.

- Dried papaya seeds, ground to a paste, or raw papaya slices gently rubbed on the affected area, then washed, is an excellent remedy.

- *Terminalia chebula*: This fruit is rubbed with a little vinegar on a coarse grinding stone. The fluid thus obtained should be applied on the skin.

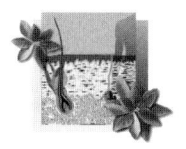

WHITE PATCHES ON THE SKIN

White patches appearing on the skin spell fear for most people as they assume they have a socially unacceptable disease, leprosy. This is very rarely so.

Causes and symptoms

White patches on the skin can be due to a number of causes. One of them is a fungal infection called tinea versicolour. These are small, distinct, irregular-bordered, light spots. They may or may not itch, and any of the treatments suggested for fungal infection will see it fade away.

However, there is a another type of white spots seen in some children, on the exposed surfaces of the body, especially discernable in dark-skinned people. These cause no problem and often disappear, unnoticed. Some are of the opinion that they are caused by intestinal worm infestations or a calcium deficiency in the diet. It may or may not be so, but in some cases de-worming helps.

Patchy depigmentation of the skin is a problm for many people. It often starts with the hands, feet, face, and around the eyes or lips. This is a genetically passed-on trait, which occurs in some generations in some people, and passes over others in the same family. Apparently, stress is the triggering factor which causes this problem, or having inferior plastic goods in constant contact with the skin, e.g., cheap, rubber or plastic slippers, bra hooks, watch straps, cheap plastic frames of spectacles. There is no permanent cure for this affliction in any system of medicine. However, the progression of depigmentation is arrested by medication in some cases. This disorder does not cause any problem or dysfunction other than its unsightly appearance. It is called leucoderma or vitilago.

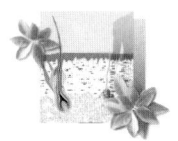

Remedies

The herbal remedies given below may or may not show results, but they can be tried out.

■ Finely powdered, dried peepul-tree bark: A teaspoon of this should be mixed with coconut oil and applied on the skin.

■ In the early stages, the application of juice extracted from fresh fig leaves is efficacious.

■ Drinking 1-2 tablespoonful of bitter gourd juice daily often has an effect on the stress-relieving mechanism. It enhances the positive functioning of the psycho-immunary axis.

■ Black cummin-seed paste with a little natural vinegar is also beneficial.

■ Drink a cupful of milk with half a teaspoon of sandalwood powder added to it. It a known fact that the application of sandalwood paste is a protection against harmful radiation from the sun's rays. Maybe this is an offshoot of this belief. Sandalwood fragrance helps those who practice meditation. It may have a stress-relieving, psychologically-soothing effect.

■ The application of a paste made with a tablespoonful of powdered radish seeds and a teaspoonful of vinegar is effective.

BODY ODOUR AND SMELLY FEET

With changing times and drip-dry clothes have also come deodorants and anti-perspirants, to give that 'everfresh, whiffing past you fragrance'. Alas, all these hide is the smell of sweat, a natural excretion from the skin!

In warm weather cotton is the most skin-friendly fabric. This goes for socks too.

Remedies

■ Bathe daily, using a mild soap and water, especially in summer. Soap can be replaced by natural ingredients available in the kitchen. These will not deplete the skin of its natural oils, but actually preserve and nourish it while removing dry, dead skin.

■ A paste made with a tablespoonful of coarsely ground lentils, yoghurt and a few drops of lime juice makes a good body scrub.

■ Dried apricot peels, or dried orange peels, can be ground fine and bottled. These peels should be dried in the shade. Apricot peel has oils similar to bitter almond oil. This oil is used in making some skin creams. The oil obtained from orange peel is used to make some beauty soaps. Its oil is extremely volatile and has a deep cleansing action. Being from the citrus family, it is rich in vitamin-C. Its low pH value helps maintain the mild acidity required for healthy skin. Add a teaspoonful to your lentil-oatmeal body scrub. Those of you who have a dry skin should use apricot peel, whereas an oily skin benefits from orange peel. Do not mix them, but use them as needed. The peel should be used on alternate days or twice a week. They leave one with a clean and fresh feeling.

■ Any flower whose fragrance appeals to you and makes you feel fresh can be used to prepare an infusion, e.g., rose, jasmine, lavender, marigold, geraniums, or sandalwood shavings. A cold infusion added to the final rinse after your bath will leave you in a 'I am on top of the world' mood for the rest of the day. Or stitch a small muslin bag, fill it with your favourite herb/ flowers, fasten with a rubber band and place it in the bath water 5-10 minutes before a bath. The water absorbs the essential oils and when you bathe, a thin film stays on the skin surface.

■ Make sure you have a clear stomach. Treat any tendency to constipation. (Look up section on constipation.)

■ Those who wear shoes and socks for long hours and have a tendency to perspire more than normal usually suffer from smelly feet. Every evening wash your feet well, dry and air them—leave them uncovered for a while. Once or twice a week soak them in neem water for 8-10 minutes. Always clean the webs of the toes well and dry them. Half a teaspoonful of powdered alum added to a litre of water and used to rinse the feet acts as an effective astringent and reduces sweating effectively. Sweating is a normal excretory function of the body, so do not unnecessarily interfere with it. If the sweating seems abnormal, consult a physician. Acacia leaves, pomegranate leaves, or ground tamarind flowers also make excellent anti-perspirants.

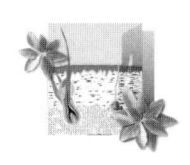

LEPROSY

The white patches on the skin that one needs to worry about are those where there is associated loss of sensation. A depigmented patch that does not pain when pricked with a pin, or does not feel the sensation of a feather lightly touching it, needs to be investigated. This is likely to be leprosy—a communicable yet fully treatable disease by allopathic means. Leprosy is caused by a bacterium. Its spread is through contact with skin lesions or nasal discharges, and it has a long incubation period. Constant close contact with a patient for over five years might show the disease surfacing after another 3-5 years. Hence, this is a totally preventable disease, if suspected, detected and reported in time.

In some cases, the area affected by leprosy may become hyperpigmented and thickened, and the underlying tissue damaged. Loss of sensation causes inadvertent injuries to the affected areas, as there is no sensation/ feeling. These injured areas have necrotic tissue and debris.

Remedies

- Folk knowledge advocates the use of the fresh sap from the soft bark of the neem tree—a teaspoonful—taken daily for six weeks. The sap should also be applied on the lesions.

- Lesions should be soaked in neem water for 40 minutes daily. Neem bark/leaves are equally efficacious.

FRECKLES/ BLEMISHES/ SPOTS

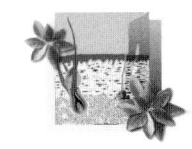

Some people have small pigmented spots on the face, which occur naturally, and are not caused by infection.

Causes and symptoms

These are caused by a natural disposition to an excess deposition of melanin on scattered areas, often triggered by exposure to sunlight. Some people get these in their growing years, but women often get them in their forties, that is, the pre-menopausal years. These have no relation to actual menopause, but since they seem to appear in the fourth decade or later, they may have something to do with aging. These pigmented spots are called freckles. Blemishes are another kind of skin discolouration which are caused by exposure to cold winds. Circumscribed blemishes on the face are called spots.

Remedies

Make the following combinations for face packs, which can be applied on the face and washed off when dry:

- For normal skin, soak a tablespoonful of lentils for a few hours. Drain off the water and grind them to a coarse paste. Add a few drops of fresh lime juice to the paste.

- To a tablespoonful of honey, add a few drops of fresh lime juice and a pinch of salt.

- Dry orange peels, powder and store them. To use, add rose water to make a paste. Helps remove dry skin scales and cleanses the skin.

- Wet a jambul seed in water and rub it in a circular motion on a smooth, washed stone. Collect this watery residue-filled liquid and apply it on individual blemishes, spots, pimples, etc. Let it dry. Wash it off with water. Do this for a few days.

- For a dry skin, apply a paste made of a tablespoonful of dry pumpkin seeds and a little olive oil.

- An expensive face pack for dry, aging skin is to soak 4-5 almonds overnight. Skin and grind them and make a paste with a little milk.

- For oily skin, soak a tablespoonful of lentils overnight. Drain off the water.

Grind it to a paste with a little yoghurt or milk. Keep the paste on till it dries. Wash it off with warm water.

■ Make a paste of gram flour, yoghurt and a pinch of turmeric. If the skin is dry, replace the yoghurt with fresh cream.

■ Use fresh buttermilk as a face pack, followed by a warm water rinse. It reduces the oiliness of skin predisposed to pimples and acne.

■ Using sesame-seed oil for a facial massage reduces dryness.

Note: These packs should not be used daily. Use them once or twice a week. Some skins are sensitive to gram flour and may develop a rash. Hence, when using it for the first time, use just a little bit. Sometimes, using it on the arms and legs may not cause a reaction, but on the face it does.

PIMPLES/ ACNE

The bane of adolescence, the 'wonder years', is a very common skin disorder called acne.

Causes and symptoms

A blockage of the oil glands present at the base of the hair follicles causes the formation of pustules, normally referred to as pimples. Practically all teenagers suffer from a pimple or two, and some from acne, in a mild or severe form. It does not spare either sex, though in boys it often appears in a more vicious form. Acne is a consequence of a juggling of pre-puberty and puberty sex hormones. Once these settle down, the acne disappears or limits itself to an odd pimple appearing during the pre-menstrual phase. This hormonal imbalance causes over-production of oily secretions by the sebaceous glands that lie at the base of the hair follicle. Under normal conditions, the secretion is just enough to keep the skin healthy. But, over-secretion coupled with dirt, dust and grime from the environment makes an ideal breeding ground for micro-organisms. When a bunch of pustules rupture and coalesce, the base hardens, and nodules form. If these are now scratched, as teenagers so often do to try and quickly get rid of them, reinfection occurs, healing is delayed, and fibrosis and scarring take place. Some drugs also predispose or actually cause acne, e.g., steroids, anti-epileptics, tranquillisers and immuno-suppressives.

Remedies

■ Strict cleanliness is the key word as far as acne is concerned. Wash the skin well with soap and warm water, followed by a rinse with cold water. Pat dry and ensure that the skin is clean, devoid of any creams or make-up.

■ Avoid using harsh medicated scrubs, skin-peelers or cleansing agents. Better still, use a herbal cleansing-cum-soothing face pack that will soften and cleanse the skin without abrading it.

■ Washing the skin with fresh buttermilk, and then rinsing it well with warm water maintains the pH balance of the skin, thereby making it a difficult proposition for bacteria to thrive.

■ A jambul seed, dipped in water and rubbed on a smooth-surfaced stone or chopping board, will yield a thin paste. Apply this selectively only on the pimples. Let it dry. Wash it off with warm water.

■ A face pack made with either gram flour or lentil powder and half a teaspoonful of turmeric can be used on alternate days. If you are sensitive to gram flour, replace with lentil powder.

Make a thin paste of one-fourth of a teaspoon of nutmeg powder and a teaspoonful of sandalwood powder with a little milk. Apply. Let it dry. Leave it on for 10 minutes and then wash it of. Nutmeg has volatile constituents that have a sedative, benumbing effect. There are exposed nerve endings at the base of the damaged tissue, which carry the pain/ itch fibres. Myristicin, a volatile ingredient that is an active principle in nutmeg, probably acts upon these. So the pimple does not itch, and the person does not touch it. This also prevents auto-infection or re-infection. Sandalwood has anti-microbial properties because of the presence of an ingredient, santalol. This combats the bacteria/germs that have caused the inflammation. The action is so potent that termites do not attack sandalwood per se. It is, by itself, also an anti-inflammatory agent.

Another remedy using nutmeg and sandalwood is to take a pinch of these two ingredients and add a pinch of powdered black pepper to it. Use milk to make a thin paste. Apply locally 2-3 times a day for 2-3 days. The nutmeg and sandalwood act as soothing agents. As explained earlier, sandalwood also has an anti-microbial and anti-inflammatory action. This is further potentiated by a substance, pipperine, in pepper, which has an anti-bacterial as well as antiviral and antibiotic action.

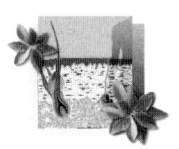

- Take a teaspoonful each of lightly roasted mustard seeds, dried orange peel powder and *buchanania letifolia*. Grind these together with a little water and apply on the face. Let the pack dry. Wash it off with warm water.

- Holy basil-leaf juice or neem-leaf juice can also be applied on the pimples for three or four days. This will heal the pus-filled pimples. Holy basil has very potent anti-inflammatory properties and also some antibacterial action. Neem has a very specific action on micro-organisms that attack the skin. The pulp of the neem fruit can also be applied with a little buttermilk or milk.

- Dried orange peel, moistened and gently rubbed over the skin stimulates circulation and acts as a very gentle scrub to get rid of dried scabs.

- Scars left by healed pimples or acne lesions can be got rid off by using a pack made up of a tablespoonful of lentils, ground with a teaspoonful of milk, with a pinch of camphor added, and a few drops of hot, fresh ghee. Mix well and apply. When it dries, gently rub it off and wash with warm water.

- Pureed tomatoes: Take one-third of a cup of pureed tomatoes. Add fine oatmeal and a teaspoonful of honey to make a paste. Apply this as a thick mask. Leave it on for 10-15 minutes and wash it off with warm water. This cleanses and clears blocked pores.

- Fuller's earth: Take one-third of a cup of finely powdered Fuller's earth, and add a tablespoonful of fresh potato juice to it. This makes a good deep-cleansing mask. Wash it off with warm water and then splash cold water on the face.

- Fresh garlic paste applied on individual pimples gives antimicrobial protection to the lesion and helps it to heal .However, it may cause a little burning as its sulphur-containing volatile oils are very pungent. Its bactericidal effects are more potent than carbolic acid. Use initially on a single pimple, as in some cases the irritation caused may be too much to bear.

- Grind a teaspoonful of dried onion seeds with a little milk. Add half a teaspoonful of fresh lime juice and apply it on the pimples. Leave overnight. Wash it off in the morning.

- To a cup of unheated fresh milk, add a tablespoonful of fresh lime juice and let it stand for a couple of hours. At bedtime, wash your face well with water, and pat it dry with a clean, absorbent towel. Now apply this milk on your face. Do not wipe, but let it dry. Leave it on overnight, and wash it off in the morning. Carry out this treatment once a week for a few weeks. It ensures that the acidity of the skin is maintained at a healthy pH, which dissuades bacterial growth.

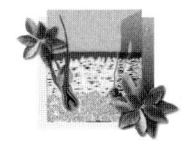

■ Take a tablespoon of oatmeal, mixed with enough fresh yoghurt to make a paste. Add a pinch of turmeric and apply it on the face. Leave it on till it dries. Wash it off with warm water.

■ A paste of fresh, tender leaves of lime or neem, with a large pinch of turmeric, also makes an effective anti-bacterial face pack.

■ Finely ground cinnamon with a little fresh lime juice, applied on the pimples, has an antiseptic and astringent effect. This can be used frequently.

■ Fresh fenugreek-leaf paste is cooling, soothing and curative for acne. Apply at night and wash it off in the morning. Fenugreek-seed tea, taken off and on, helps purify the blood and keeps infection at bay.

BLACKHEADS

The oil ducts lying at the base of the sebaceous glands get blocked with oil, the daily dust and grime of the environment, and result in blackheads. Some people try and remove them by pricking them with a needle, pin or tweezer. These are incorrect and unhygienic measures, and will only make the blackheads worse.

Remedies

■ Regular washing of the skin and applying any of the cleansing packs suggested for pimples, e.g., the dried orange peel, tomato-puree and onion-seed packs will all help in cleansing the pores and softening the skin. Gentle yet firm pressure applied to the base of the blackhead with a clean cotton bud will extrude the grimy contents. Wash the face again with cold water and pat it dry.

■ Using a yoghurt-lentil mask twice a week will keep the skin clean and soft.

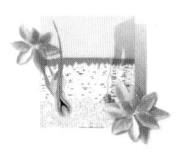

■ For pimples, acne and blackheads, when present together, or just as a preventive measure for those prone to them, try the papaya pack. Take the pulp of an over-ripe papaya, mash it well and apply it on the face. Avoid the eyes. Gently rub it into the skin. Some will come off. Remove this, and without washing, apply a fresh layer. Leave it on for 15-20 minutes. This takes some time to dry. When it is not fully dry, wash it off with lukewarm water, and dry the skin well with a slightly rough towel. Now massage a few drops of sesame-seed or coconut oil into the skin. Leave it there for an hour. Wash it off with warm water. This will get rid of the oiliness. Do not use soap. Continue this treatment for 3-5 days. Repeat after 6-8 weeks. It will keep the skin glowing and healthy. There are certain substances in ripe papaya pulp which dislodge deposits and grimy concretions, cleanse and heal unhealthy tissue, and stop bleeding. Coconut/sesame-seed oil acts as a soothing agent and an emollient, and prevents scarring of the healed lesion. Wherever there is healing, the natural elasticity of the tissue is lost, because elastic fibres are replaced with fibrous tissue which contracts, leading to the puckering of acne scars. The natural oils have substances that work at various biochemical levels to help maintain maximum elasticity in the tissues, to prevent puckering and early wrinkling.

SHINGLES/ HERPES ZOSTER

Shingles/herpes zoster is the name given to a skin condition that occurs as a result of a flare-up of a dormant chicken pox virus lodged in the nerve roots of a patient who has had the infection in childhood.

Causes and symptoms

This skin condition occurs in later years, often a result of a debilitated physical condition or a stressful life, that causes the body's immune system to be depressed. The immune system may also be depressed due to certain immunosuppressive drugs such as corticosteroids, anti-cancer agents or immune disorders like AIDS.

The virus replicates and spreads along the distribution of the nerve root, causing skin lesions that appear like blisters and cause a sharp burning pain.

Shingles usually appear in later years, but children too may be susceptible. The lesions can appear anywhere—on the trunk, chest, shoulder, side of the face, eye, etc. It is normally one-sided but can appear on the other side too. When it attacks the eye, it can cause permanent damage and blindness due to scarring and subsequent opacity of the cornea in the affected eye.

Remedies

The best treatment for this condition are anti-viral drugs. However, herbal remedies may help, complementing orthodox treatment.

Eat plenty of fresh fruits, vegetable juices, especially carrot juice, as the body needs large amounts of beta-carotenes, bioflavonoids and vitamin-E to combat the virus.

ALLERGIC RASHES/ URTICARIA

In allergic rashes and urticaria, red patches appear on the skin. There is a whitish area in the centre of the patch and a gradually increasing, red, inflamed circular periphery.

Causes and symptoms

These patches are a reaction to some food, or contact with an allergen—a substance the body does not recognise as its own, or does not take to, and reacts with a violent physical manifestation. These red patches itch with a burning intensity, swell up and cause acute distress. Sometimes they subside after a couple of hours. At times active medical intervention is needed, as the discomfort tends to overwhelm the patient to the point of his going into a state of shock, that can have disastrous results.

Urticaria can also occur due to bee and wasp stings, even mosquito or bedbug bites, and sometimes, exposure to severe cold winds. Shellfish, tomatoes, eggs, chocolate, nuts, milk and food additives are proven culprits which can cause urticaria.

Remedies

■ To your bath water add 2-3 tablespoons of powdered rock salt or soda bicarbonate. This will relieve the itching to some extent.

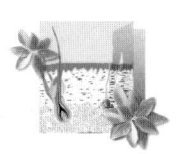

■ Mix 1-2 teaspoons of fresh ginger juice with a teaspoon of honey in a glass of water and drink it at 2-hourly intervals till the itch disappears. Do this for not more than a day.

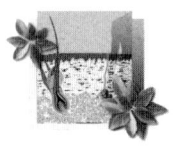

- One or two teaspoonsful of fresh mint juice with honey is also very efficacious.

- The application of a thin layer of sandalwood paste has a soothing effect.

ECZEMA

Eczema is a non-specific term that refers to an inflammatory presentation of a certain skin disorder of known or unknown origin.

Causes and symptoms

In eczema there is redness, localised swelling, vesicle formation, rupture of this vesicle, and subsequent moist or actual weepy, watery discharges from the lesions that leave behind raw surfaces. There is also an intense desire to itch. The person scratches the affected area, and the condition gets worse. Th symptoms are often worse and aggravated at night.

There are various theories which suggest that this disorder has a constitutional / genetic predisposition. Other studies claim that a disturbed metabolism, nutritional allergies, stress, autoimmune dysfunction, emotional upheavals, precipitate an inherent predilection to present with this very distressing picture. This condition has two distinct presentations—a dry eczema where there are dry lesions with a tendency to itch, and wet, weepy lesions that make it difficult for a person to function normally. According to ayurveda, the accumulation of toxins in the body, and their inadequate elimination, or a blockage in their elimination, leads to eczema.

Remedies

- When there is a fresh patch of dry eczema, applying freshly-made ghee (from cows's milk butter only), and washing the area well a number of times, relieves the itch.

- Dry the peel of a watermelon, the large variety that has a deep green skin and bright red pulp with black seeds. Burn the dried peel to an ash. Take a spoonful of this ash and add enough warm coconut oil to make a paste. Apply this on the eczematous patch.

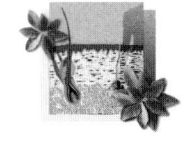

- Muskmelon: This remedy can only be tried in summer when this fruit is in season—a 40-day diet of eating only sweet muskmelons should be undertaken under the supervision of a qualified and experienced ayurveda. Fresh juice taken daily is also beneficial. This can be taken as a beverage, and also used for local application.

- Use a diluted neem decoction for washing the weepy lesions twice a day, then pat them dry.

- Apply a paste made with a tablespoon of fresh, crushed neem leaf and a teaspoon of turmeric powder. If possible, use a fresh turmeric root. Add a spoonful of sesame-seed oil. Apply once a day.

- Boil a tablespoon each of mango-tree bark and acacia-tree bark in half a litre of water. Filter and use this to wash the eczematous patches. The water should be warm enough to act as a fomenting agent, but not hot enough to burn. Pat dry and apply fresh ghee.

- A decoction made with the bark of the peepul tree can be used to wash weepy, eczematous lesions. It has an astringent as well as an antibacterial action. It acts against staphlococcus aureus and E.coli, which are the cause of many secondary skin infections. The decoction also contains tannin, which heals ulcerated lesions.

- Take a piece of sandalwood and rub it on a smooth stone or chopping board with a few drops of water. Collect a tablespoonful of the paste. Use a nutmeg to do the same, and collect a tablespoonful of this liquid too. Mix the two together and apply it on the skin. Nutmeg blocks the pain and sandalwood soothes the itching of inflamed tissue. This remedy should only be used sometimes to relieve extreme distress. Nutmeg gets absorbed and may cause toxic symptoms if the accumulated dose is too much. Use sparingly.

  A pinch of camphor can be substituted for nutmeg. Camphor is also derived from a tree—*cinnamomum camphora*. When used topically, it has an antipruritic effect. However, this too can have a toxic effect, so it should be used sparingly.

- Auto-urine therapy: This much-maligned therapy (raised eyebrows by orthodox medicine practitioners!) has a prominent place in ayurveda for the treatment of certain disorders. For eczema, the patient is advised to go on a totally vegetarian diet—eating no animal products at all, including butter, ghee, eggs, etc. As far as possible, the stress is on eating raw, fresh, easy-to-digest foods. Seven days after starting this diet, the early morning specimen of urine should be collected and applied immediately on the eczematous lesions. Leave it on the skin for 20 minutes, and then wash it off with normal, clean water. No soaps or detergents should be used. The patient should not have any alcohol, take drugs or smoke during this treatment. This treatment should be continued for a week or ten days—by then the eczema will heal. The therapy can cease, but the vegetarian diet should continue for a while, till healing is complete. A check should be kept as cooked and other foods are introduced, one at a time, and the effect watched, so as to eliminate the eczema-precipitating food factor, if at all it is caused by a food constituent. This remedy is a proven one, related to me by people who have suffered from this complaint and have resorted to this remedy. They have been symptom-free for more than 8-10 years. They had been on allopathic treatment for many years, but had found no relief. We, who are practitioners of modern medicine, must remember that there are a number of drugs still being selectively extracted from the urine of pregnant mares, human placental tissue and other body fluids.

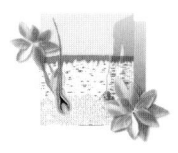

■ Lastly, for all skin troubles, make sure the patient has no constipation and eats a nutritious diet, rich in green vegetables and fruits. Avoid tea, coffee, alcohol, sugar, white-flour products and processed foods. Go off junk foods.

PSORIASIS

Psoriasis is not an uncommon disorder. It is the result of a genetic error, where the cell-division phenomenon goes berserk.

Causes and symptoms

It is a benign condition identified by the appearance of dry, circumscribed silvery scales on bright red patches, generally on the soft inner sides of the elbows, knees, crotch, forehead or scalp. However, there is no hard or fast rule. They can appear anywhere on the body. Though unpleasant-looking (no skin condition is actually pleasant to look at

NUTMEG

Botanical name:
Myristica fragrans

Description and uses: The nutmeg tree is an evergreen, yielding a hard, aromatic and spheroidal seed. This seed is grated and used as a spice to flavour a variety of cuisines all over the world. It has a strong but pleasing fragrance, with a slighty bitter and aromatic taste. Nutmeg also has several less-known medicinal uses. It is used to alleviate general weakness and debility, anaemia, toothache, flatulence and diarrhoea.

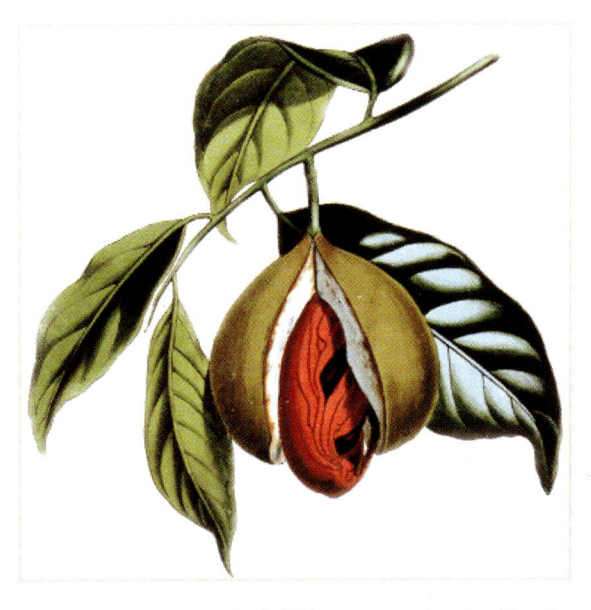

other than a flawless complexion), it is not infectious.

Usually the skin renews itself in four weeks' time, that is, new cells form in the dermis layer and keep maturing and moving upwards from the innermost to the outermost surface layer. In psoriasis, there is a short circuit, and this happens in about four days. So there are too many new cells struggling to find a place in the outermost layer, which has not yet shed itself fully. This results in raised areas or plaques that have new red cells, which are itchy. The new cells will now age and die like the old cells, but there are just too many of them. They are dry, like silvery scales being shed. This phenomenon is not consistent. Sometimes the disorder is at its peak, at other times there is a remission or a normal phase.

Why this genetic error occurs is not known. Whether it actually has a genetic pre-disposition is also not certain. What triggers off this malfunction is also not known. Since there is no known cause, the cure is also not certain. It is palliative, and only relieves the distressing symptoms. There are many cures advocated for it, some of them more specific than the others. Which therapeutic modality will work on whom, how well it will work, and whether it will work at all, are all unanswered questions.

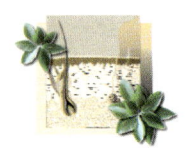

Remedies

With all the known, lesser known and just-being-tried treatment modalities in the orthodox, modern medical set-up, here are some word-of-mouth remedies that seem to have survived generations of changing medical systems. They lessen discomfort and control, if not really cure, exacerbations.

■ Try and avoid stress and stressful situations—a tall order indeed!

■ Switch to a diet rich in raw, vegetarian food, especially vegetable and fruit juices.

■ Avoid milk and milk products, citrus fruits, alcohol and tobacco.

■ Increase intake of fibre, wholemeal wheat and wholegrain cereals

■ An oatmeal bath soothes the skin irritation and itching. Put 500 gms oatmeal in a thin cloth bag and soak this in the bath water. Squeeze it gently in the water after it has been submerged in it for some time. Remove the bag, and now immerse the patient in the bath. Pour the water over the area with the lesions. After this treatment, bathe the patient, using a mild soap-nut solution instead of soap.

■ Cook on a low flame fresh drumstick-leaf juice mixed with sesame-seed oil in equal quantities, till the water evaporates. Cool and apply as a salve.

■ The decoction of a handful of drumstick leaves added to bath water is soothing and prevents secondary infection of the skin.

■ Half a cup of bitter gourd juice, taken daily during the acute phase of the disorder, provides ample vitamin-A and C, besides being active medicaments for healing lesions.

■ Select a cabbage with very green leaves—the greener the leaves the better. Separate the leaves and remove the thick central vein in each. This will effectively divide it into two. Wash the leaves and wipe them dry. Flatten each on a heated non-stick griddle and apply them one by one on the lesions, interlacing one leaf over the other. Bandage lightly with a cloth. This acts as a soothing compress. Cabbage leaves contain S- methyl-methioninine, which promotes healing of the skin and also relieves pain.

■ Boil a handful of marigold flower heads in a litre of water. Cool and use these as swabs on the skin lesions. Bathe with soap-nut solution.

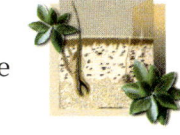

■ Lesions can be washed with a litre of water to which a tablespoonful each of fresh lime juice and neem-leaf juice has been added.

■ Use fresh jasmine-flower paste to apply on the lesions as a soothing salve.

EXTERNAL ULCERS

External ulcers are a result of infection in a break in the skin, an excavation at the base of a local lesion produced by the sloughing of necrotic inflammatory tissue.

Remedies

All the remedies suggested earlier for the treatment of boils or pimples will bring relief and heal external ulcers.

■ For the treatment of old chronic ulcers, the sap (milk of raw papaya) is efficacious. Wash the ulcer area with warm water. Cut a raw papaya and scoop out the pulp. Mash it well and apply just enough to cover the ulcerated area. (Avoid putting it on normal skin). Let it dry. Then apply a light bandage over it. Next day, wash it off. Repeat again. The ulcer will heal within 4-5 days. Do not overdo this application.

■ The sap of the banyan tree is also used to clean chronic ulcers that discharge pus.

■ Ulcers resulting from underlying diabetic diathesis are difficult to treat. Anti-diabetic treatment has to be followed meticulously to yield and sustain any results. (Look up section on diabetes.) For the diabetic ulcer, roast a semi-ripe brinjal. Remove skin and seeds. Mash the pulp. Add a pinch of camphor and apply the mixture on the ulcer. Repeat for 3-4 days. The ulcer will heal, provided the diabetic diet and treatment is strictly followed.

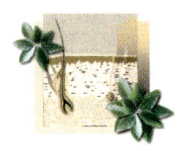

VARICOSE VEIN ULCERS

Varicose vein ulcers are extremely painful and cause great distress. They need urgent remedial care and treatment.

Causes and symptoms

Poor circulation in the legs causes distension of the veins. There is pooling and stagnation of blood, as the one-way valves in the veins are not functioning well, impeding the return of blood to the heart. Initially, changing position and elevating the limb relieves the condition, but soon it becomes a permanent distention, disrupting fresh blood supply to the tissues in the area. This causes itching and a wound—and an ulcer forms. A varicose vein ulcer is typically pale, discharging in the centre, itchy and red on the periphery.

Remedy

■ For temporary relief, bathe the ulcer with an infusion of marigold, sage, geranium, neem or holi basil.

Note: Do not treat varicose vein ulcers at home. It can be dangerous. Consult a doctor immediately. There is a strong possibility of dislodging debris that could result in emboli travelling to distant vital organs, with a disastrous outcome..

WARTS/ VERRUCAS

Warts are small, hard growths, originating from the epidermal or uppermost layer of the skin. Warts can occur anywhere on the body. When they occur on the soles of the feet, they are called verrucas.

Causes and symptoms

Of the various theories regarding the etiology of warts, the most accepted one is that a particular virus is to blame. They can be very painful on the soles, otherwise they cause no problem except for their unsightly appearance. Warts can appear and disappear without reason. However, if touched or pricked with a pin, some can spread. So, unless they interfere with functioning, or press on an underlying nerve, causing pain, do not try removing them. If any of these complaints arise, its time to consult a physician.

Remedy

- Onion juice, raw potato juice, or the milky extract of fresh figs, applied several times a day on the wart, for at least a week to ten days, sometimes helps.

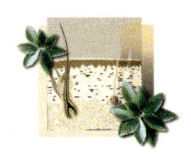

EXCESSIVE TANNING OF THE SKIN

Being out in the sun can give one a particularly unpleasant-looking dark tan, and getting rid of it seems an impossible task.

Remedies

- Rub the rind of a lemon on the skin. Leave it on for 15 minutes and wash it off.

- Prepare a mixture of fresh lime juice and rose water in equal quantities, the paste of a few fresh fenugreek leaves, and a few drops of glycerine. Apply this mixture on the skin and leave it on for an hour. Wash it off with warm water, followed by a cold-water rinse. Dry the skin well and see it sparkle

- Use regularly a spoonful of fresh lime juice with a teaspoonful of honey and a few drops of olive oil as a massage mixture on the face before having a bath. It leaves the skin clear and glowing.

Note: *Any of the face packs suggested in the section on blemishes will also clear a troublesome tan.*

PRURITIS / ITCH

A disagreeable sensation that compulsively excites the desire to scratch is called pruritis or itching. Just under the skin are minute nerve endings that carry the sensation of touch, pain, heat and cold. It is believed that the fibres that carry the sensation of pain also excite the desire to scratch. This happens when the stimulus is not sharp or potent enough to be interpreted as pain. A lesser stimulus causes the desire to scratch, whereas a stronger stimulus causes pain—but why the desire to scratch arises without any apparent stimulus is a mystery.

LIME

Botanical name: *Citrus acida*

Description and uses: The lime tree is small and prickly, with ovate-oblong leaves and small white flowers. The fruit is smaller, greener and more acid than a lemon. It is rounded, and has a smoother and thinner rind. Lime juice was formerly given to sailors to prevent scurvy on long voyages. It is a rich source of vitamin-C, and is used in the manufacture of citric acid. The pulp, juice and rind of the fruit are extensively used to prepare herbal remedies for anaemia, nausea and vomiting, hypertension, mouth and throat problems, ear problems, indigestion, flatulence, colic, constipation, diarrhoea, jaundice, piles, a burning sensation when passing urine, excessive urination, arthritis, chapped lips, body odour, freckles, acne, psoriasis, varicose vein ulcers, pruritis, hair problems and morning sickness in pregnancy.

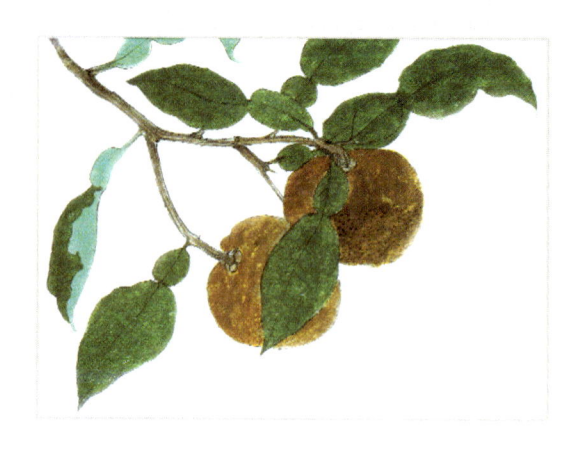

Causes and symptoms

Most skin disorders have a common presentation, the desire to scratch, for which there are many causes—local irritant stimulus due to insect bites, mosquito bites, mite bites, fungal infection or even eczema. General causes include systemic disorders like diabetes mellitus, nephritis, jaundice or drug reaction. Here the stimulus is internal, due to a metabolic/ systemic dysfunction along some other pathway. Other causes include allergy to chemicals, soaps, perfumes, artifical heating, cold weather or low humidity. Healing of skin lesions causes fibrosis, because the elastic fibres are replaced by fibrous tissue which stretch when there is swelling or pressure in the area. This too causes an itch.

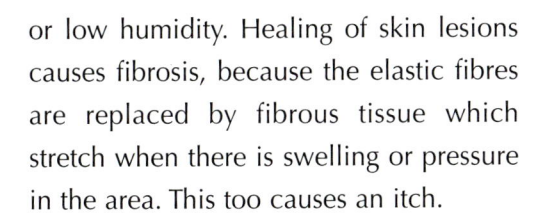

Remedies

■ Equal quantities of fresh tomato and coconut juice, mixed and applied on the itchy area, will bring relief.

■ A tablespoonful of split red gram ground to a paste with fresh yoghurt and applied locally for 4-5 days is effective.

■ Grind dried orange peels to a paste with a little water. Apply for a week.

■ Have a daily massage with warm sesame-seed oil.

■ Sprinkle lime slices with rock salt. When dry, grind in a dry grinder and store. Take one-fourth to half a teaspoonful once or twice a day (not for hypertensives).

■ Grind the root of a bitter gourd and make a paste. Apply locally.

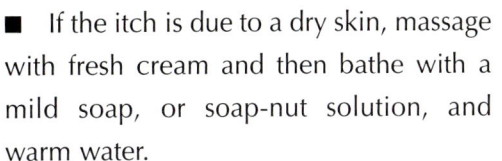

■ If the itch is due to a dry skin, massage with fresh cream and then bathe with a mild soap, or soap-nut solution, and warm water.

■ Drink fresh buttermilk with a little grated ginger for seasoning.

■ For an itchy scalp, a regular weekly massage with warm olive oil, sunflower or sesame-seed oil will take away the dryness.

■ Make your own shampoo for an oily, itchy scalp. Whisk an egg and gradually add this a tablespoonful of fresh orange juice. Add half a cup of soap-nut decoction and mix well. Apply this mixture on the scalp and tie up your hair. Leave for 10-15 minutes and rinse out thoroughly with warm water till the hair is absolutely clean.

■ Soap-nut decoction: Take a handful of soap nuts. Remove the skin and discard the seeds. Boil this with a glassful of water. Let it cool. Mash the boiled skins and then strain/filter. Your decoction is ready.

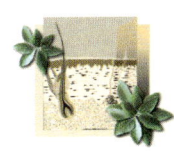

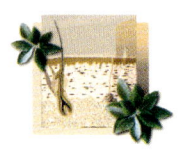

SOME PROBLEMS RELATED TO HAIR

Hair loss, lustreless hair, thinning hair, falling hair, baldness, premature greying and dandruff are the most common hair problems.

Causes and symptoms

The cause for most of these problems are incorrect diet and stress. Of course, some causes are related to genetic tendencies, systemic diseases and the side effects of drugs taken for some other condition, e.g., chemotherapy for cancer. Whatever the cause, these simple home remedies will not cause any harm. They can only help.

Remedies

■ Boil a handful of fresh neem leaves in a litre of water. Simmer for 4-5 minutes. Let it cool. Filter and use as a rinse after washing hair with a soap-nut decoction. This will prevent dandruff as well as hair loss. It will also remove any lice present.

■ Massage the scalp with warm coconut oil twice a week, followed by wrapping a damp, hot towel on the head. Wash after half an hour with a soap-nut decoction.

■ Shoe flower, or the Chinese hibiscus, also known as *hibiscus rosa-sinensis:* Heat a cupful of coconut oil and fry 8-10 flowers in it till they are black and charred. Cool the oil. Filter and keep aside to use as a hair oil.

■ Dry and powder curry leaves and lime peel. Take equal measures of powdered curry leaves, lime peel, fenugreek seeds, mung dal and shikakai. Mix and keep aside. Use this as a shampoo. Wet hair and apply the mixture—the amount needed depends on the thickness and length of the hair. Leave it on for a few minutes and then massage it into your scalp. Rinse with warm water. This leaves the hair clean, soft and shiny.

■ Fry a handful of coarsely pounded curry leaves in a tablespoonful of hot coconut oil till it is charred. Let it cool. Grind and apply to the scalp. Leave for an hour and then wash it off. Use the shampoo given above.

■ Pure almond oil is expensive but very nutritive for the scalp. It prevents hair loss.

■ Some people like to wash their hair very often. Do not use chemical shampoos. Apply fresh fenugreek paste on the scalp and hair and leave it on for 15-20 minutes. Wash it off with plenty of water. Do not use any shampoo.

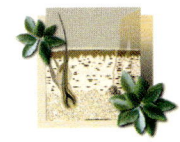

LICE

Lice are tiny parasites that infest the scalp, trunk, armpits or the pubic areas. They cling to the hair roots, so they inhabit all the hairy areas of the body.

Causes and symptoms

Lice infestation occurs because of poor personal hygiene, close contact with people who have lice, using infected combs, sharing infected clothing, even sitting on sofas or sleeping on beds used by infected people. It is easy to spot head lice, but body lice are difficult to locate unless there is a massive infestation. Lice can spread infections such as typhus, relapsing fever and trench fever.

Lice are usually spotted because they cause itching where they lodge. They lay eggs, which become nits that are easily visible as little white eggs sticking to the hair. Nits are difficult to dislodge. Even if lice are picked and removed, nits mature within a week, and the cycle restarts.

Remedies

■ The best remedy for lice is neem leaf. Make a paste of a handful of neem leaves and apply it to the scalp with a little coconut oil. Leave overnight and wash/shampoo in the morning. Repeat this application 2-3 times.

■ Garlic paste and fresh lime juice applied at night and washed off in the morning also gets rid of lice. Repeat for 2-3 days.

■ Apple-cider vinegar, or mashed apple left to discolour, should be applied to the scalp and left for half an hour. Massage well, and then shampoo. Onion juice or finely mashed onion paste can also be applied to the scalp, left for 3-4 hours, and then the hair shampooed. Repeat for 3-4 days.

■ Custard apple seeds can be dried and powdered, mixed in coconut oil, and applied to the scalp. Leave it on for 2-3 hours and then wash off or shampoo with a soap-nut decoction.

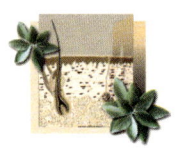

WOUNDS

Small cuts and wounds should be washed well in running water to remove dirt and grime. If the wound is very deep, use a neem-leaf or fig-leaf decoction to wash it. Let the wound dry on its own for a while before dressing it.

Symptoms

If there is much bleeding, apply a pressure pad made with a clean folded handkerchief or cloth. Wounds that are large and badly lacerated need to be attended to by a doctor for suturing. Suturing should not be delayed for more than 6-8 hours. For small wounds, herbal home remedies will suffice.

Remedies

- Fresh garlic juice diluted with an equal amount of water, or coarsely crushed garlic paste made with water, can be applied, especially if there is a suspicion of the wound being infected.

- Apply the fresh juice of the aloe leaf, or its pulp, on the wound and bandage it.

- Neem-leaf paste with turmeric, in equal quantities, is efficacious.

- For festering wounds and sores, use tender papaya-leaf paste as a poultice. Remove it after it cools and apply a clean dressing with turmeric paste.

- A tablespoonful of liquorice powder, a spoonful of honey and a little ghee can also be used for dressing wounds. It does not stick.

- A paste of ripe bitter gourd mixed with a teaspoonful of sugar is effective.

- When a dressing sticks to a wound, apply the medicament, and then cover it with a warmed betel leaf or a thin banana leaf smeared with coconut oil, and bandage it.

BURNS

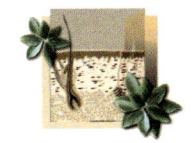

Burns are the result of tissue injury caused to the skin by its being exposed to excessive friction, intense heat, chemicals, electricity or radiation.

Causes and symptoms

Burns can damage various layers of tissues, and the treatment depends on the severity of the injury. The seriousness of the condition of the burnt area depends on the total surface area of skin involved and the depth of the tissue injured. Survival depends on the total surface area involved. The greater the surface area of the skin involved, the more dangerous the burn. Large surface areas mean more blister formation, and hence, more swelling and fluid loss. This results in shock that is life-threatening.

Note: *Treat only minor burns at home that are not more than a hand's width in their surface area, and are not deep. Chemical and electrical burns may not extend over a large surface area, but damage deeper tissues. For anything more than minor surface burns, seek medical care at a hospital with an intensive-care burn unit.*

Remedies

■ Immerse the burnt area in tepid water or slightly cold water for 5-10 minutes. This reduces the heat and relieves the pain.

■ If blisters begin to form, do not prick them. If the burn is caused by a corrosive agent, or there is cloth sticking to it, do not try and remove the cloth. Take the patient to a doctor.

■ A scald burn may form a blister and the area hurts every time something touches it. The remedies above can be applied to soothe the pain. If the blister bursts, do not apply there remedies. Look up section on burst blisters.

■ Sometimes there is no blister but just a local redness due to singeing. Take the soft, tender leaves of the banyan tree. Grind them to a paste, add a little fresh ghee made from cow's-milk butter, and apply it on the skin.

■ A paste of the soft, tender leaves of the *zizyphyus jujuba* tree is also very soothing. It has an astringent action that prevents blister formation.

■ An ointment made with powdered cloves and honey prevents infection.

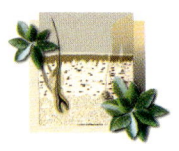

■ Sometimes, after a burn has healed, the area becomes lighter than the surrounding area, or may even appear nearly white. This is because the underlying layers of skin that have the melanin-producing cells are destroyed, and only scar tissue remains. Honey, with its natural enzymes, energises the regenerating layers and the melanin-producing cells. It ensures that the skin regains its natural colour.

■ If burns are caused by an acid, wash in running water and apply bicarbonate of soda dissolved in fresh buttermilk, or made into a paste with fresh yoghurt.

■ If burns are caused by caustic alkali or lime, wash with running water, followed by a rinse with a glass of water to which a teaspoon of vinegar has been added. Then cover with a beaten egg white, or the paste of ground chalk mixed with linseed oil.

For minor burns which you feel do not need medical attention:

Apply mashed banana on the burn. This will prevent blister formation.

∽

Henna-leaf paste or pomegranate-leaf paste is very soothing and takes away the pain.

∽

Raw potato juice or grated raw potato can be mashed and applied on the burnt area.

∽

Apply some honey locally.

CORNS/ CALLUSES AND ROUGH HEELS

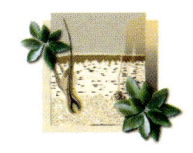

Corns, calluses and painful heels with hard rough skin, sometimes with painful cuts, are a result of persistent rubbing, pressure and friction on the skin.

Causes and symptoms

These problems are caused by ill-fitting shoes or wearing no shoes, walking and working on particularly dry, dirty, pebbly soil. Corns per se are harmless, but because they hurt when pressure is put on them, people have a tendency to shift their normal weight-bearing line/axis to avoid pain. This causes pressure on areas of the sole which are not meant to take the extra pressure, which results in more corns, at times even orthopaedic problems. Some people also have an inherited tendency to abnormal callus formation.

Remedies

- In areas prone to calluses, like the elbows, hands, knees, ankles and heels, rub the area gently with a rough cloth or a pumice stone while bathing. Pumice stone, or the dried skin and fibrous skeleton of ridge gourd (*luffa acutangula*), do a fine job of removing dried dead skin, dirt and grime.

- Those prone to corns or dry heels should, after a hard day's work, soak their feet daily in a basin full of very warm water to which a little shampoo or soap-nut solution has been added. Soak for 5-10 minutes till the water cools. This not only relaxes one after a hard day at work, but also prevents corns from forming, or at least makes them less painful. Dry the feet well and massage in some oil—coconut oil, sesame-seed oil, olive oil, castor oil, or fresh milk cream, butter or ghee, any greasy base will soften and soothe the skin. Soak once again to remove excess oil and dab dry.

- A poultice of shredded lemon peel, raw tomatoes or fresh pineapple helps soften corns or hard skin.

- Persistent hardcore corns need to be surgically removed.

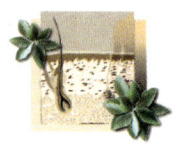

BITES AND STINGS

Man lives in an environment which is inhabited by many other living beings. As long as we live in harmony and do not get in their way, other creatures will not usually harm us. Yet, the stress and congestion in our living conditions are such that various insects or animals may bite us. Long before the advent of anti-sera and vaccines, man survived these episodic hazards. Here are a few tried and tested remedies used by people who do not have access to specialised medical care.

ANT/ BEE/ WASP OR HORNET STINGS

Of all these stings, the bee sting is the one to beware of. By itself a sting may not cause a problem. But multiple stings, like when a beehive falls on one, can cause a life-threatening situation. Some people are also allergic to bee venom.

Causes and symptoms

When a bee or wasp bites, it injects its venom just under the skin surface. There is a sharp pain, localised swelling and redness. The pain may last for a couple of hours, or even a day or two. Swallowing a bee will result in the bee stinging the vocal cords. This results in a swelling inside the throat, which causes discomfort in breathing that could have a fatal outcome. A bite in front of the ear can cause the venom to be injected into the facial nerve that lies just below the skin surface, causing local facial paralysis. Multiple bee stings cause cells in the area to break up and disintegrate, releasing destructive debris and metabolites that are carried away by the circulation, to be filtered out by the kidney. The kidney tubules and blood vessels get overloaded and blocked, leading to irreversible kidney failure, resulting in an overall shutdown of other systems too—which can, and often does, have a fatal outcome.

Note: So, if you are stung by many bees or wasps, rush to a hospital. Do not try a home remedy. For a single bite try the following remedies:

Remedies

■ Wash the area with cold water and place an ice cube on it. Then apply a little salt to it. Rub it in, but not hard enough to push the sting in. Carefully scrape off the skin with a blunt knife and remove the sting with a tweezer. Do not squeeze it as that will cause the residual venom to be re-injected into the skin.

■ A bee sting or ant bite also feels better if a paste of baking soda and water is applied on it. Parsley juice or honey smoothed on the swelling will also relieve irritation.

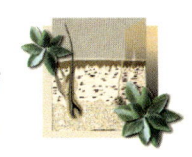

MOSQUITO BITES

Mosquitoes are a menace in tropical climates, and their bite is painful and causes itching.

Remedies

■ Rubbing camphor, balm or Vicks Vaporub on the area relieves pain and stops the itch.

■ Mashed garlic is effective, and baking soda and honey paste will also relieve the pain. However, garlic will not let the area get infected. Lemon juice application helps too.

■ To get rid of mosquitoes, flies and bed bugs, dry orange peels and store. Place the orange peel in a pan with glowing hot coals. These insects do not like the fumes. Dried neem leaves, eucalyptus leaves or omum seeds have a similarly unpleasant effect on them. Keep crushed garlic tied in a muslin bag and hung up in a corner where mosquitoes congregate.

SPIDER BITE

Small spider bites are harmless, but the fiddle back and black widow spider can cause trouble. The fiddle back spider is light brown in colour. It is a large spider with a dark brown/ black, violin shape on the back of its head. It is found in colder climates.

Causes and symptoms

When this spider bites, there may be mild discomfort and not much else. But in some cases, red spots form on and around the site of the bite, soon becoming bullae. These bullae, in a day or two, become ulcers with a deep bases. There is inflammation, fever with chills, muscular and generalised joint pains. A generalised swelling may also occur.

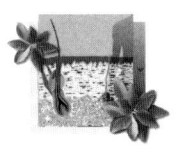

Remedies

- Cold compresses and elevation of the bitten part relieves the pain of a fiddle back spider bite.

- Using a hot water bottle relieves the pain of a black widow spider bite

- Folk remedy: Make a paste with dried, unripe mango-peel powder and water. Apply on the bite/ wound.

Note: *The body is usually able to cope, but not always. Hence, should these changes occur, shift to a hospital immediately.*

The black widow spider is a warm-weather spider, usually found in dessert areas. The female of the species is deadly. It is a really large spider. The body measures about a centimetre , with legs that are 4-5-centimetres long. Its big body has a red hour-glass shape on the back. This spider is vicious and will bite at the least provocation.

Causes and symptoms

The bite produces a momentary, severe cramping pain. Then shivering starts, with intermittent sweating, and the pain begins. There is nausea, vomiting, headache, laboured breathing, with the abdominal wall becoming rigid like a board. The symptoms often mimic a perforated appendix or an ulcer pain. An acute presentation may at times appear like a heart attack.

Note: *If bitten by a black spider, rush to a hospital fast. Timely help is needed to combat impending cardiac/ respiratory failure.*

TICK BITES

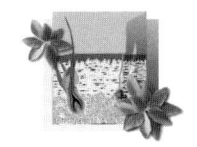

Those of us who keep dogs as pets are aware of the troublesome nuisance of tick infestation in dogs. By themselves ticks may not be a problem, however ugly they look, climbing all over the walls where the pet normally sits.

Causes and symptoms

What is worrying is when a tick bites you or your dog. The local reaction is redness and itching in the area. If the tick is not removed, it stays stuck to the area and continues to suck blood. Its saliva secretes a toxin that affects the nerves. In some sensitive cases, this toxin causes slow paralysis—there is a feeling of weakness, restlessness and irritability because one is not sure what is wrong. As paralysis sets in, different systems are affected. There may also be respiratory distress. Timely removal of the ticks and symptomatic supportive treatment reverses the problem. Absence of fever or any violent active symptoms are responsible for delay in treatment, but one should remember that the toxin can take some time to reveal its full effect.

Remedies

■ All ticks must be removed from an animal. Herbal tick baths with neem decoction are available, but you can make your own.

■ Individual ticks can be removed by dabbing kerosene on them and then lifting them off with a tweezer. Incomplete removal may cause the sting to remain. This results in a local inflammation and the formation of a nodule. Scratching this results in a secondary infection, or the nodule starts increasing in size, giving rise to the mistaken diagnosis of a tumour.

TICKS ARE ALSO VECTORS FOR DISEASES LIKE TULAREMIA, TYPHUS AND LYMES DISEASE. IT IS IMPORTANT TO DE-TICK YOUR PET BECAUSE TICKS HAVE THE POTENTIAL OF SERIOUSLY HARMING YOUR HEALTH.

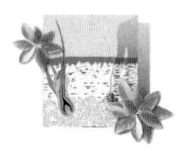

DOG BITE

A dog bite is a dangerous thing. Dogs are the most common pets, and they should be protected against rabies and other diseases. A dog bite or scratch must be immediately washed and cleaned with soap and water, as the rabies virus can gain entry into the body even from a minute abrasion. The virus is transmitted through a dog's saliva. If the dog is a stray, it is obviously not immunised, and it is vital to seek medical help. The virus can lie dormant for a few hours to a couple of days, but it is actively multiplying all the time. It should be immediately neutralised at its site of entry. No time should be lost.

Remedies

■ Finely ground red chili powder/ paste applied immediately on the wound neutralises the virus. The wound does not get infected, and heals fast. This remedy really hurts, and the pain may cause shock.

■ Asafoetida, powdered fine and dusted thickly on the bite, apparently draws the infection out. It has a pronounced astringent effect and absorbs local moisture and the virus.

■ An application of fresh onion juice and honey is another remedy.

Note: *These are only stop-gap remedies and should be tried if the dog is immunised or can be kept under observation. However, any bite in the head and neck area, or a large bite elsewhere, should be medically attended to. THERE ARE ONLY THREE KNOWN SURVIVORS OF RABIES WORLDWIDE.*

LEECHES

Thin, needle-like leeches abound in wet, marshy areas. They latch themselves onto the skin and suck blood. At one time they were put to use to suck out pus and blood from infected wounds!

Remedy

■ Drop a pinch of salt on the leech head where it is stuck to the skin. It will fall off without causing pain. Do not try to pull it off, as its mouth parts can break off and remain embedded in the skin, causing an ulcer-like lesion.

SCORPION STING

Scorpions are small creatures with eight legs and an uplifted tail and have a near-lethal sting. These creatures prowl around at night, or stay hidden in dark corners, under stones, logs, undergrowth, crevices, etc. They are in colours that are an excellent camouflage for them.

Causes and symptoms

The sting of a scorpion carries venom of different potencies, depending on the species. It causes a burning sensation that spreads in waves all over the body. This may last for a few hours and then pass off. But at times, the reaction may be very severe, and systemic changes like increased heart rate, sweating, restlessness, nausea, vomiting, etc., may occur. Very severe reactions can be fatal.

Remedies

- Calm the patient and immediately apply a cold compress on the bite area.

- Crush lavender leaves, apply on the site and bandage lightly.

- Crush mint leaves and apply locally. Simultaneously, drink a teaspoonful of fresh mint juice or eat mint leaves.

- Sweet potato leaves should be ground to a paste and applied locally. The dried tuber can also be ground and applied.

- Tamarind seed: Rub a tamarind seed on a hard surface to crack the outer brown covering. Remove the covering. Apply the white kernel on the sting. It will absorb the venom from the site and also the sting.

- Apply fresh onion juice locally.

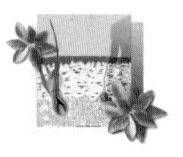

SNAKE BITE

When a poisonous snake senses someone approaching, it makes a characteristic hissing sound and moves away, a non-poisonous snake just slithers away.

Symptoms

The bite of a poisonous snake induces a feeling of intense weakness. The patient does not become unconscious immediately. If he or she becomes unconscious at once, it is probably due to the shock of the bite. The poison spreads through the circulation.

COBRA/KRAIT OR SEA SNAKE BITE

Symptoms

The effects are evident within ten minutes to two hours of the bite. Even though the wound is very small (in some cases the bite is practically invisible), there is intense burning at the site of the bite. The poison does not let the blood clot and it starts oozing from the bite within 2-3 hours. There is hardly any swelling at the site, but there is a slowly progressive feeling of weakness, unsteadiness on the feet, and a creeping paralysis sets in. The patient finds it difficult to speak and feels sleepy, though he or she does not lose consciousness. Breathing becomes laboured and death is due to respiratory failure.

Note: *The critical time to treat a cobra or krait bite is to do so within a few hours to two days. It takes two days for the patient to actually succumb to the bite. So timely intervention, taking the patient to a hospital, will save his life.*

VIPER BITE

Symptoms

In a viper bite, the wound marks are visible and a swelling appears at the site. There is intense burning and the swelling increases to about 8-10 cms. A fluid starts oozing out of the bite. The poison attacks the circulatory mechanism of the body and the pulse becomes thready. The patient feels cold, the skin becomes clammy, and bleeding occurs from the nose, stomach and internal organs. The crisis takes place within 6-12 hours. The patient dies within a few days. So timely intervention is the need of the hour.

Note: *For an undiagnosed snake bite, whether it is poisonous or not, seek medical help within 6-10 hours. You may be able to save the patient.*

Remedies

■ Tie a tourniquet above the site of the wound and immobilise the area.

■ The folk remedy is to suck the venom out. It can be done. The venom only enters the blood through the circulation. So if there are no wounds, cuts or injured raw surfaces on the mucous membrane inside the rescuer's mouth, the poison can be sucked out. It is, however, rarely recommended or done today. If the venom is swallowed by mistake, it will not cause any harm, as snake venom is a protein and will be acted upon by enzymes that break down proteins. Modern medical concepts discourage this practice. However, villagers in tribal areas in India, where doctors fear to tread, still suck out the poison and are apparently none the worse for it.

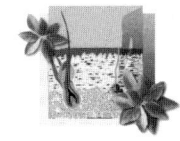

■ In an emergency, place crushed lavender leaves on the bite area and tie a bandage. The essential oils of lavender neutralise the venom to some extent and minimise damage

■ A pinch of powdered alum added to a teaspoonful of fresh ghee should be applied to the bite area. Alum soaks up the venom and the ghee delays its absorption.

■ The bark of the flame of the forest tree: Equal quantities of crushed bark and ginger are ground together and administered to the patient. This is supposed to control the bleeding and haemorrhage, and is believed to be an antidote to the action of the venom on the patient's system. It is a remedy used by people living in forest areas in South India, but has not been tried out under medical supervision.

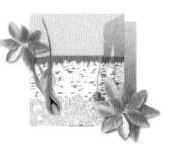

POISONING

Any substance that causes harm to the body by simple contact with the skin, or by ingestion, inhalation or injection, is a poison. This can occur accidentally or be done intentionally.

The fastest way to remove a poison that has come in contact with the skin is to simply wash the skin thoroughly with soap and water. All contaminated clothing should also be removed as irritant oils, chemicals, etc., can spread to other parts of the body by continued contact.

If the poisoning is due to contact with a plant, do not put the contaminated hand on the face, eyes, mouth or the genitals. These areas are extremely sensitive, and local irritation, rashes and swelling, as well as systemic effects like breathing difficulties and scarce urination may occur.

Remedies

- If the poison has been injected, the best way to get rid of it is to make the patient vomit. However, ingestion of oily substances or caustic chemicals can make this an extremely dangerous procedure, as while being vomited these substances cause immense damage to soft tissues.

- If a poisonous plant has been ingested, make the patient vomit by putting a finger into the throat and initiating the gag reflex—to expel the poisonous substance out forcefully by vomiting.

Note: *It is difficult to have a blanket treatment modality for all ingested poison cases, as there are some specific antidotes for each.*

- For ingestion of a caustic, corrosive poison, make the patient drink diluted milk with charcoal.

- For corrosive liquids ingested, give 1-2 glasses of milk. Do not add charcoal to this. It can cause mechanical obstruction.

- For ingestion of paint thinner, nail-varnish remover, petroleum products, give milk and charcoal.

- For ingestion of insecticides, fungicides, pesticides, give charcoal and milk.

- For suspected arsenic poisoning, as with rat poisons, garden pesticides, etc.,

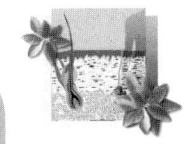

THE UNIVERSAL ANTIDOTE FOR INGESTED POISON IS TO MAKE THE PATIENT DRINK TEA WITH CHARCOAL. PREPARE A WEAK, LUKEWARM TEA. MIX POWDERED CHARCOAL IN IT, AND MAKE THE PATIENT DRINK IT. THE CHARCOAL ABSORBS THE POISON, WHICH CAN THEN BE DE-ACTIVATED. CHARCOAL IS GIVEN IN THE PROPORTION OF 1 GRAM PER KILOGRAM OF BODY WEIGHT. IF IT IS NOT IMMEDIATELY AVAILABLE, BURNT TOAST WILL DO.

give the patient 2-3 glasses of milk to drink, to which add 3-4 beaten egg whites, or a weak starch solution, e.g., cooked rice water or a thin flour solution.

■ For sewer-gas poisoning, if the victim is still breathing, bring him into the fresh air and give him plain soda water to drink. This neutralises the initial acidic reaction of the absorbed gases.

■ Induced vomiting only helps in poisoning due to barbiturates, pesticides and rodenticides.

■ For cyanide poisoning, do not induce vomiting, or give stimulants like tea, coffee, etc., as they only worsen the condition by drug interaction.

■ Ingestion of methylated spirit or adulterated liquor: This causes cramps, dizziness, headache, confusion, convulsions, cloudiness of vision and permanent blindness. The sooner the antidote is given the less the chances of permanent side effects. If there is delay in treatment of more than 12 hours, the effects become irreversible. (Actually, symptoms of toxicity only begin to surface after 12 hours). However, cramps and nausea are the first warning symptoms, so action should be initiated immediately. The simplest antidote is to administer a large peg of whisky. Whisky has ethyl alcohol, which will compete with methyl alcohol for absorption and metabolism. So it is safe to give this and rush the patient to a hospital.

Many health problems such as hyypertension, diabetes, allergies, to name a few, are stress-related disorders. To keep them at bay, lead a healthy and disciplined life, and try to keep away from unnecessary tension—this is the prescription for a stress-free and pleasant life.

■ STRESS-RELATED DISORDERS

The fast pace of modern life has brought in its wake high levels of anxiety and depression. Not that they did not exist earlier, but life was simpler, and just getting housework done, looking after home and hearth, cocooned in the serene surroundings of nature, eating simple wholesome meals, with no labour-saving devices, the body was exercised naturally and it remained fit. Man lived in harmony with nature. Even if problems occurred, the remedies were taken from nature.

Modern lifestyles are often synonymous with junk food, addictions, sedentary lifestyles, and a tendency to isolate oneself—be lonely in a crowd. There has also been a rise in the level of competition for scant resources and a race to get the best and the most for oneself. Tensions begin in families, right after a couple get married, about whether to have a child or not, and then whether to have one or more children, as moral pressure from 'elders' to have a family 'in time' and so on carries on. Too soon after the child enters the world, begins the often harrowing experience of school admissions. Once in school, there is excessive pressure of studies, then the stress one has to undergo for admission into college, then work, and jumping jobs to get the best—it goes on and on. The five vices, as enumerated in the Hindu scriptures, *kaam, krodh, moh, lobh, ahankar,* meaning excessive indulgence in carnal pleasure, anger, lust, avarice and possessing a a inflated and massive ego, all these lead to problems in life. One never seems to find happiness, which is a state of mind. Now it has been scientifically proven that many of our physical complaints are caused by our lifestyles. However, the intricacies of a discussion on anxiety, depression, lifestyle is beyond the scope of this book

Remedies

■ Get out of the rat race. Learn to live life as pleasantly as possible on a daily basis. Save for a rainy day, but don't work as if you are looking out for the rain all the time. As long as your work does not cause you to harm anyone in thought, word or deed, there is no reason to fear the future. Live with an attitude of gratitude, in harmony with nature. Work by all means, but take time to reflect and relax. Learn to meditate. Look within yourself and be content. Take daily ups and downs in your stride, and do not let them become obsessions and terrifying monsters, so that they interfere with your sleep and day-to-day normal functioning. Have a nutritious and wholesome diet. Have meals on time with the family—TV dinners consisting of snack foods, and watching violence on the screen, is not conducive to healthy digestion. Take regular exercise—a daily walk (even a kilometre or so) contemplating on nature as you walk past a garden, see flowers, trees, anything pleasant, is relaxing.

■ Have a relaxing massage once a week, with stress-relieving, soothing herbs immersed in the oil used for the massage. Stress-relieving herbs are holy basil, fennel, geranium, thyme, marigold and sage. Soothing herbal teas are made from holy basil, mint, nutmeg, cinnamon, fenugreek, fennel and lemon. These teas should not be had on a daily basis, only when needed.

■ Fresh lime juice and honey or fresh orange juice every morning is beneficial.

■ Eat plenty of greens, salads, vegetables and fruit.

■ Always have a light breakfast before you go out to work.

■ Drink plenty of water.

■ Cut down on tea, coffee and aerated drinks. A drink once in a while is stimulating. As a routine, however, it becomes an addiction and causes dependence on it.

■ Smoking is definitely a NO.

■ No man is an island—an evening spent with friends, or a picnic once in a while, is a nice way of putting daily cares out of your mind, especially in nuclear families.

THYME

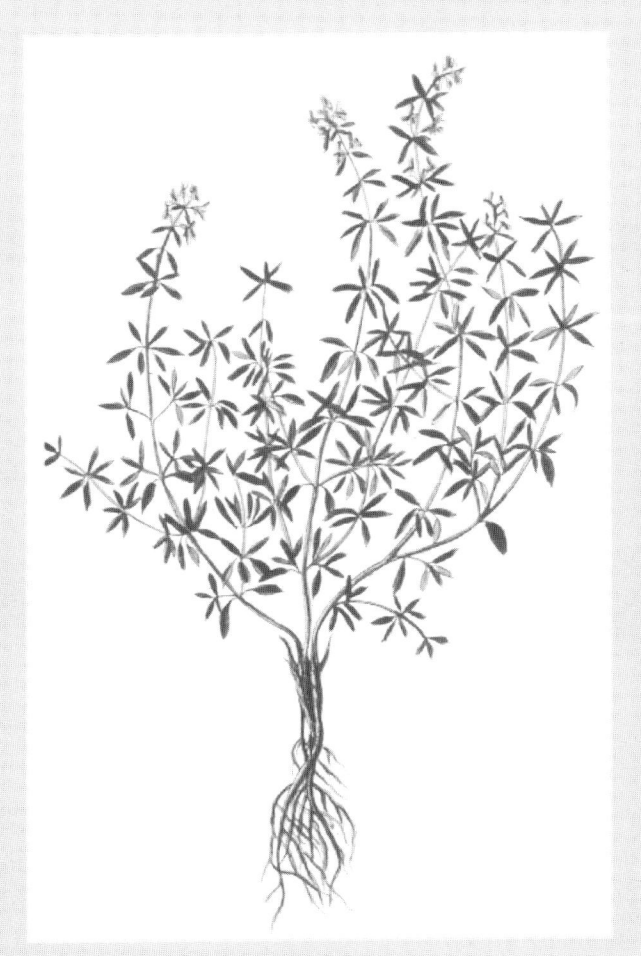

Botanical name: *Thymus vulgaris*

Description and uses: The leaves of the thyme plant have an agreeable aroma and a pungent taste. The fragrance of the leaves is due to an essential oil it contains, which gives it its flavouring value for culinary purposes, and is also the source of its medicinal properties. The leaves are used fresh or dried to treat headaches, sore throats, flatulence and colic.

There are several causes for sexual debility and weakness—some are actual physical problems, but many are psychosomatic in nature. In order to live a healthy, normal and contented life, these disorders need to be tackled and treated without delay.

SEXUAL DEBILITY AND WEAKNESS

Sexual debility or weakness implies a number of sexual issues such as lack of desire, inability or inadequate ability to perform the sex act to completion, lack of satisfaction on completion of the act, and inability of the partners to mutually satisfy each other.

A sexual act will only be fulfilling if it is performed under the right circumstances— sex between mutually consenting, sexually-aware adults, within the sanctions and accepted norms of society, in natural, happy and healthy surroundings. Over-indulgence in sex, without external excitatory influences, can itself be a cause for debility. This subject per se is too large and complicated to be treated lightly. It is outside the scope of this book. However, some simple remedies are suggested. They enhance desire and performance, but not necessarily the sperm count. None of these remedies should taken for more than 4-5 days.

Remedies

■ Have with hot milk 5-7 black peppercorns crushed to a powder and mixed with honey.

■ Have half a teaspoon of long pepper powder with 6-7 crushed almonds in a cup of milk at night.

■ Soak overnight 6-8 almonds. Next morning, remove the skins and grind the almonds to a paste. Have this with a glass of hot milk to which a pinch of turmeric has been added. Add palm candy or sugar to taste.

■ Replace turmeric in the previous remedy with a pinch of saffron dissolved in a tablespoon of cold water. Add this to the hot milk. Saffron is more potent when it is not boiled in the milk but added to it.

■ Have a *paan*, (betel leaf) with almond paste and a pinch of saffron once a day.

■ Onion seeds, powdered: Take half

a teaspoonful with sugar or honey 2-3 times a day.

- Onions, cooked or uncooked, are known to excite the senses.

- Have once a day two cloves of garlic, crushed and sautéed in ghee. Use garlic in your cooking.

- Asafoetida is used in daily Indian cooking. It has a rejuvenating effect. Fry one-fourth of a teaspoon in ghee. To this add fresh latex – half a teaspoon of sap taken from the banyan tree. Slice a ripe banana and smear the sap on the surface. Put the slices together and eat it in the morning for a few days.

- Dry Chinese hibiscus flower buds and powder them. To a teaspoonful of the powder, add a cup of warm milk with a teaspoonful of honey, and have it twice a day. Avoid non-vegetarian food.

- Mix a pinch of nutmeg powder with a teaspoon of honey in a scrambled half-boiled egg. Eat it at night.

- Soak a teaspoonful of wheat grains, poppy seeds and fenugreek seeds separately in water at night. Grind all three to a fine paste and drink with hot milk daily for a few days.

- Have two teaspoons of fresh Indian gooseberry juice with two teaspoons of honey daily on an empty stomach in the morning. This can be taken for 4-6 weeks.

- Have a teaspoon of pomegranate-seed powder with milk once or twice a day for 4-5 days. It is constipating, so too much should not be taken.

- Have a teaspoon each of sesame seeds and jaggery (often made into a sweet) once a day for 4-5 days, or have it occasionally.

- Omum seeds and the kernel of tamarind seeds, in equal quantities, should be lightly fried in ghee. Then grind and store them. A teaspoon of this powder, taken with a tablespoon of honey and a glass of warm milk at bedtime is beneficial.

- Herbal tea made with fenugreek seeds is an effective remedy.

- Half a teaspoon of fresh ginger juice with a scrambled half-boiled egg and a teaspoon of honey should be taken at bedtime.

- Fry about two cups of fresh drumstick leaves in a tablespoon of ghee with half a teaspoon of black pepper powder. Cook lightly for 5 minutes. Have daily with your food for 4-6 weeks.

- Boil two tablespoons of drumstick seeds in a cup of milk. Strain it and have it for 4-6 weeks.

- Crush a tablespoonful of drumstick flowers and boil them in a cup of milk. Strain and have at bedtime.

- Asparagus root is exceptionally good for the female reproductive system. Simmer a teaspoon of the dried root powder in a cup of milk with one-fourth of a teaspoon of ginger powder. Take off the fire, add finely chopped dates (3-4 of them), and have daily for a few days.

- *Cynodon dactylon:* Your common lawn grass is also called Bermuda grass. This is a three-bladed grass. Grind a few stems and leaves to a fine paste. A teaspoon of the paste with milk – one cup—with sugar to taste should be taken daily at night for 2-4 weeks.

FOR WATERY SEMEN OR A LOW SPERM COUNT

These are fairly common problems and need to be treated. Apart from conventional treatment, the following remedies are often efficacious:

Remedies

- Dry some tender banyan-leaf shoots in the shade. Powder them. A teaspoon of this powder with a teaspoon of jaggery should be taken with a glass of milk daily for a week or ten days.

- Or, instead of banyan-leaf buds, take the fresh, tender buds of the peepul flower. Dry and powder them and have them in the same way as the banyan-leaf shoots.

Both these belong to the same family, and their action is to thicken the semen and also prevent its early expenditure, i.e., prevent early ejaculation, pre-ejaculation or emission.

Most women face some kind of gynaecological problems at different stages in their lives. Be they period pains or other disorders connected with menstruation, childbirth, infections of the genitals, and so forth, they require urgent remedial treatment so as to ensure a healthy, trouble-free life.

GYNAECOLOGICAL PROBLEMS

Gynaecological disorders are sometimes the bane of a woman's existence from the time she is a young girl. However, this does not have to be so. Prompt and correct remedial care and treatment solve most of these problems.

PERIOD PAINS OR DYSMENORRHOEA

Painful menstruation or pain during the time of the monthly periods is called dysmenorrhoea. Congestion in the pelvic organs and ovulatory cycles are the causes of dysmenorrhoea during the early years of womanhood. Dysmenrrhoea which starts in the later years may be related to pelvic infections, fibroids or other gynaecological conditions.

There are certain chemicals called prostaglandins that a woman's uterine lining produces every month. These help the uterus to contract and discharge its tissue and tissue fluids, which were formed to make the lining conducive for a fertilised ovum to embed itself. For some unknown reasons, when these prostaglandin levels are too high they cause cramps.

Remedies

■ Holding a hot-water bottle on the abdomen will give temporary relief.

■ Decrease your salt intake a day or two before your periods are due. This helps excess fluid to be easily discharged by the kidneys, thus relieving pelvic congestion.

■ Take a long leaf of aloe vera. Wash it well and put it into a mixer to extract the juice. Strain and filter this juice. Take a tablespoon of this with honey 2-3 times a day for 4-5 days. It has an added laxative effect. So vary the dose as required. Make fresh juice every day.

■ Papaya aids menstrual flow. Have a large bowlful daily during your periods. Papaya also has a laxative action, so monitor the amount taken. It is supposed to have oestrogen-like prapriaties.

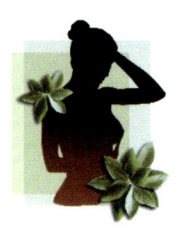

■ A cupful of carrot juice drunk once a day is also beneficial.

■ Carrot and parsley soup help in combating period pains.

SCANTY PERIODS

How many days a menstrual period lasts, how much is the flow during the duration of the periods—it all varies according to individual patterns. As long as a woman has her periods every month, regularly, the cycle being anywhere between 26-35 days, it is normal. The bleeding may be for two, three or even six to seven days. The rhythm and duration of the periods is person-specific, depending upon a woman's individual hormone settings. Sometimes the cycle may change after a D&C (dilatation and curretage) or childbirth. The amount of bleeding depends on the thickness of the lining shed, and the thickness of the lining depends on hormone balance, diet, exercise, emotions, stress, etc. As long as a cycle is regular, it is not considered abnormal or scanty.

Some **herbal teas** allay pain and anxiety during the menstrual periods. These are:

∽

Ginger tea: Boil a half to one inch-piece of pounded or grated ginger in a glass of water. Sweeten it with sugar or honey and have it thrice a day. You can have it hot or cold, as desired.

∽

Pound coarsely half a teaspoon of sesame seeds and drink it with a glass of hot water twice a day during your periods. This also ensures a smooth flow.

∽

Fennel tea should be made with a teaspoon of fennel in a glass of water. Boil, cool, strain, add sugar to taste if liked, and drink it.

∽

A herbal tea made with a handful of *mimosa pudica* leaves is beneficial. Any part of this shrub is good.

Remedies

These remedies should be started a day or two before the the due date of the periods, and taken for three to four days

- Ginger tea: Fresh ginger, pounded and brewed as a strong herbal tea, sweetened with honey or sugar to taste, should be taken thrice a day.

- Half a teaspoon of sesame seeds, pounded, should be taken with a glass of hot water 2-3 times a day, starting two days before the due date of the periods.

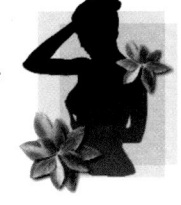

- Half to one cup of parsley or carrot juice should be taken once a day.

- Eat papaya regularly.

- Herbal tea made with marigold heads or leaves: Drink half a cup 3-4 times a day.

IRREGULAR MENSTRUATION

Irregularity in menstruation means that periods do not occur on time – that generally there is a tendency for delay.

Causes

Emotions play an important role in causing an irregularity in an otherwise normal cycle. Other causes are hormonal variations.

Remedies

- Grind 3-4 fresh hibiscus flowers. They are either red or pink, and their scientific name is *hibiscus rosa-sinensis*. Take five red flowers, grind them to a paste, and have this on an empty stomach with water for 5-7 days before the normal expected due date of your periods. These flowers have an anti-oestrogenic quality, which helps to regularise the oestrogen / progestron balance and initiate the menstrual flow in time.

- Aloe-leaf pulp: Skin 2-3 aloe leaves and collect the pulp. Boil it till it becomes brown. Cool. Mash it to make a paste. This has a slight bitter taste, so have it with water or apple juice every morning on an empty stomach for 5-7 days. The dose is a teaspoonful. This also has a purgative action, so decrease the dose if required.

- Make a decoction with a teaspoon of

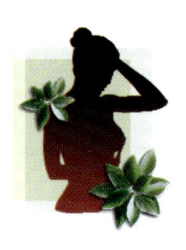

old jaggery and a teaspoon of pounded omum seeds. Have with hot water twice a day for 3-4 days before the due date of the periods.

■ Have a teaspoon of fresh holy basil-leaf juice with a teaspoon of honey and a pinch of black pepper powder twice a day for 4-6 weeks. This regularises the periods.

EXCESSIVE MENSTRUATION OR MENORRHAGIA

Some women may naturally have a heavier flow during the menstrual period than others. However, if you have excessive bleeding, which is a change from your normal cyclic routine, and the flow contains large clots, it is advisable to consult a gynaecologist. There could be an underlying problem of hormonal imbalance, polyps, fibroids, or even cancer.

Remedies

■ Coriander-seed decoction: Boil a teaspoon of coriander seeds in a cup of water till it is reduced to half. Add sugar to taste and have twice or thrice a day while it is still warm.

■ Eat banana-flower curry every day, or have it as a dry vegetable with yoghurt. Banana flower has a progestron-like substance, so it helps regularise the flow during the periods.

■ Grind fresh *bael* leaves. A teaspoonful of this paste with warm water, had once a day, is efficacious.

■ Soak 2-3 almonds in water overnight. Next morning, remove the skins and grind the almonds to a paste with 2-3 small *bael* leaves. Add a little honey and have daily. (The bael-leaf juice should be about a teaspoonful). Follow this with a cup of warm milk.

■ Have a teaspoon of Indian gooseberry juice with sugar on an empty stomach every morning. Follow it up with a glass of warm water.

■ *Mimosa pudica* grows wild throughout India. It is a thorny shrub which spreads on the ground, has small pink flowers, and its leaves close when touched. Two tablespoonsful of the fresh juice of the leaves, taken with honey thrice a day for 3-4 days will stop the bleeding.

- Asparagus tubers: Take a tablespoonful of the crushed tuber juice with sugar thrice a day for 3-4 days.

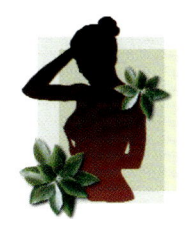

VAGINAL DISCHARGE / VAGINAL IRRITATION

One of the commonest women-specific complaints is vaginal discharge. Under normal healthy conditions, the vagina has some amount of secretion that helps keep the insides moist. At different times of the month, this secretion may be perceptible as a slight mucus discharge, or a white discharge. However, it is so little that it is not enough to stain the clothes or make one feel uncomfortable.

Causes and symptoms

Some increase in vaginal discharge takes place during excitement, sexual activity, masturbation, anxiety, in-between two periods, the day just before the period, in illness, or when one is in a rundown physical condition.

Vaginal discharge is a problem if it increases so much in amount as to stain clothes daily, if it is purulent or bloodstained, or causes itching, soreness or a burning sensation in the area.

The vaginal epithelium is kept healthy by a natural commensal in the vaginal tract called doderlein bacillus. This keeps the pH acidic, which prevents infection from setting in. Washing oneself too often with medicated soaps and detergents changes the pH, making the vagina vulnerable to infection. Being 'over clean', with the excessive use of deodorants and chemically-treated compounds, is carrying a good thing too far. Fungal infections very easily take root under these conditions. However, there may also be mixed infection and some infection contacted from sexual partners.

Remedies

- Treat anaemia or any other debilitating disorder in the body immediately.

- Eat healthy, nutritious food.

- Take care of personal hygiene.

- Crush an aloe leaf and extract two tablespoons of the juice. Have it thrice a day with honey for two weeks after the periods are over.

ALOE

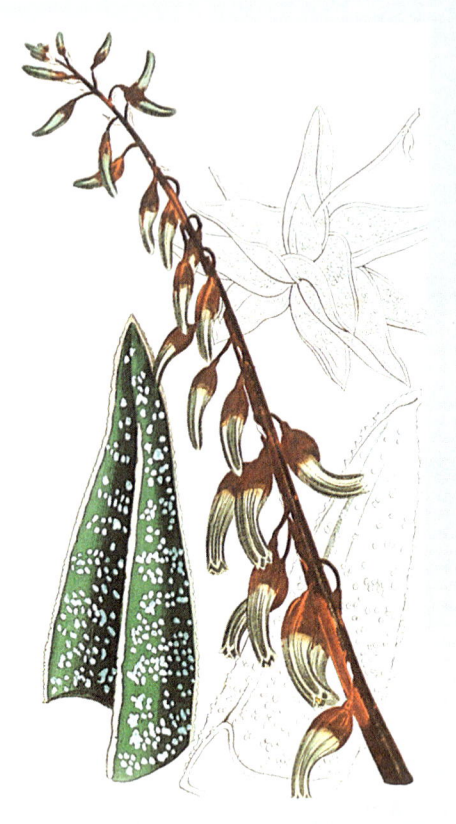

Botanical name: *Aloe vera*

Description and uses: Aloes are succulent plants belonging to the lily family and have numerous fleshy leaves. These leaves yield a gelatinous substance which is used as an emollient in cosmetics, and also as a remedy for several ailments such as head-related disorders, intestinal worms, skin problems (such as sunburn, boils, herpes, wounds) and gynaecological disorders.

■ Asparagus tubers: Extract the juice and have a tablespoonful twice a day for two weeks.

■ Hibiscus or Chinese rose-flower paste: Have the paste of 3-4 flowers with water on an empty stomach in the morning for a week.

■ Fresh henna leaves: Extract juice and have a tablespoonful twice a day for 10 days in the morning on an empty stomach, and the evening dose 4-6 hours after lunch.

■ Boil a pinchful, (6-8 threads) of saffron in a glass of water. Reduce it to half a glass. Take two teaspoonsful of this decoction daily for a few days. or dissolve a thread of saffron in a teaspoon of milk. Add half a cup of water and boil it till one-fourth remains. Have this daily.

■ Make a vaginal douche by boiling half a tablespoon each of the dry, pounded bark of the fig and the banyan tree in a litre of water for five minutes. Let it cool to a bearable temperature and use it as a vaginal douche.

■ Take a tablespoonful of the dried rind of pomegranate. Boil it in half a litre of water. Strain and use as a vaginal douche.

■ Soak a tablespoon of crushed peepul-tree bark in half a litre of hot water at night. Next morning filter it and use as a douche.

■ Make a paste of ripe *phyllanthus amarus* leaves or fruit. Have two teaspoonsful with a glass of buttermilk. If this is not available, normal ripe Indian gooseberry can be made into a chutney and had with food everyday. It is an extremely rich source of vitamin-C.

■ Take a banana, slice it and add to it a tablespoon of fresh Indian gooseberry juice with a teaspoon of honey. Have this daily for a few days.

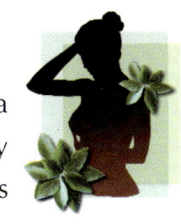

■ Eat banana flowers cooked as a vegetable, or a tablespoon of the juice of the flowers with a tablespoon of palm candy for a few days.

■ Wash and dry Indian gooseberry roots. Powder and store. Whenever there is a problem of menorrhagia or vaginal discharge, take a teaspoon of this powder, and boil it in a cup of water to make a decoction. Add sugar to taste and drink it on an empty stomach for 2-3 days.

■ For fungal infections of the vagina, when the discharge is 'curdy' white, like cheesy precipitate, with burning and pain, along with the douche suggested earlier, eat a cupful of fresh yoghurt every day.

■ Add a tablespoon of apple-cider vinegar, with honey to taste, to a glass of hot water. Drink it first thing in the morning.

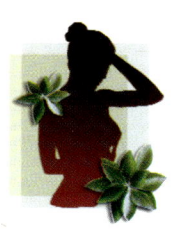

MORNING SICKNESS

A number of women complain of nausea, and some of vomiting early in the morning during the first few weeks of pregnancy.

Causes and symptoms

These symptoms usually start after the third week of the missed periods. They generally subside at 6-8 weeks, but may last for three months. Anything more than this is not normal and needs medical attention. The nausea and vomiting is a result of bio-chemical changes taking place in the body, plus the fact that certain pregnancy-related hormones are high.

Remedies

- Eating a dry toast or a cream cracker biscuit in the morning with your cup of tea will soothe the biochemical upset.

- Mix honey with some powdered green cardamom seeds. Lick it once in a while.

- Roasted gram, eaten just one at a time, slowly, allays the urge to vomit.

- Fresh orange juice with honey, orange-rind herbal tea with honey, and fresh ginger and lime tea soothe nausea.

- Eat smaller, lighter meals. Foods which have ginger, pepper, chilies, cinnamon and onion stimulate the appetite. Chew lime-peel pickles, tamarind or raw mango.

- Powder 2-3 cloves, add to a glass of hot water and simmer for 15-20 minutes. Let the mixture cool, and sip the solution off and on.

STRETCH MARKS

Pregnancy causes an increased abdominal girth, stretching the elastic fibres in the skin. Some of these fibres break and leave linear striations. These marks do not go away. To prevent this from happening, or to lessen it, gently massage olive oil into the stretched skin before a bath. After childbirth, massage with olive oil to bring back the tone of stretched muscles. However, some marks will remain.

Care of the breasts

In early pregnancy, the breasts start becoming a little fuller and the colour of the nipples darken. These changes are hormonal in nature.

Remedies

- Massage the breasts with warm olive oil before having a bath every day.

- To delay menstruation after childbirth, a teaspoon of powdered cinnamon with a cup of milk every night increases the milk produced. The hormones which increase lactation delay the onset of menstruation.

- Lightly roast, grind and bottle fennel. Have a teaspoonful after meals. It is good for digestion and ensures smooth, healthy lactation after childbirth.

LACTATION

To ensure adequate milk for the newborn, the mother's diet should include proteins such as black gram, mung, split red gram, with a little ghee and cummin seeds for seasoning.

Remedies

- A teaspoon each of powdered dried asparagus and lump sugar with milk, taken daily for 2-3 weeks in the immediate postnatal period, is beneficial.

- Have wholemeal wheat and avoid too many spices and junk food during this period. A lot of what you eat is passed on to the baby. So, if he or she has diarrhoea, it is usually caused by what you have eaten.

Congestion in the breast

If there is too much milk, there can be congestion and pain in the breast.

Remedies

- After the baby has nursed at each breast, express the extra milk. Sometimes he or she only feeds at one breast and goes off to sleep. Empty out the other breast. In a day or two, the baby will catch up and drink all he or she can.

- Do the following perineal muscle exercises whenever you remember to do so – constrict those muscles voluntarily, which you would use to stop urinating or passing stools, i.e., the urethral and anal sphincter. This will ensure that the entire pelvic floor tightens up.

Ailments and remedies at a glance

FEVER
Herbal remedies: Lavender leaves, holy basil leaves, ginger powder, Indian gooseberry, neem, coriander seeds, cardamom, cloves, cinnamon, peppercorns, cummin seeds turmeric, *bael*, fenugreek seeds mint, fennel, *swertia chireta*, sage, lime juice, honey, tamarind.

PAIN
Herbal remedies: Henna, holy basil.

HEADACHE
Herbal remedies: Marigold flowers, rose petals, lavender, lemon, orange peel, mint sage, fennel, cloves, holy basil, rosemary, *omum*, sandalwood oil, mustard oil, sesame-seed oil, coconut oil, olive oil, *marjoram*, ginger, honey, cummin seeds, mint, thyme, *terminalia chebula*, Indian aloe and drumstick leaves.

NAUSEA / VOMITING
Herbal remedies: Ginger, holy basil, honey, cloves, nutmeg, curry leaves, *bael* leaves, cummin seeds, lime juice.

HYPERTENSION
Herbal remedies: Wholegrain cereals, potatoes, avocados, tomatoes, lima beans, yoghurt, cottage cheese, sesame seeds, spinach, broccoli, chickpeas, *bael*-leaf powder, cummin-seed powder, sandalwood powder and paste, fresh green coconut water, fennel, lump sugar, Indian gooseberry, honey, orange, grape, carrot, spinach, watermelon seeds, poppy seeds, garlic, coriander seeds, holy basil leaves, grapefruit, lime juice, ginger, onion, turmeric, parsley and drumstick-leaf juice.

CONJUNCTIVITIS
Herbal remedies: Turmeric, coriander seeds, coriander-leaf juice, acacia leaves, alum, guava leaves, pomegranate juice, aloe, potato, apple, tamarind leaves, holy basil juice, neem-leaf juice, drumstick-seed oil, honey, fennel, cow's milk cream and fresh yoghurt.

NOSEBLEEDS
Herbal remedies: Coriander leaves, mango blossoms and juice of the soft kernel of a ripe mango seed.

PAIN IN THE THROAT
Herbal remedies: Bottle-gourd juice, honey, spinach juice, carrot juice, onion, cummin seeds, mulberry, dry bark of the mango tree and rose petals.

HOARSENESS
Herbal remedies: White turnip, honey, onion juice, cinnamon, cardamom, fennel, figs, almonds, hot milk, liquorice, lump sugar and black pepper.

HICCUPS
Herbal remedies: Ginger juice, honey, lime juice, pepper powder and radish leaves.

EARACHE
Herbal remedies: Eucalyptus leaves, mustard oil, sesame-seed oil, garlic, omum, holy basil-leaf juice, garlic oil, neem leaves, lime juice and pounded fenugreek seeds.

COUGH, WHEEZING, ASTHMA, BREATHLESSNESS AND CHEST INFECTION
Herbal remedies: Ghee, freshly ground black-pepper powder, drumstick leaves, hot chapattis or hot rice, dried ginger powder, cow's milk, honey, *bael* leaves, peppercorns, mustard seeds, holy basil leaves, ginger, betel (leaves), jaggery, omum, turmeric, buttermilk, cloves, onion juice, sesame seeds,

linseed, almonds, orange juice, lemon juice, fennel, Indian gooseberry powder, bitter-gourd root, fenugreek seeds, cabbage, large dried seedless grapes and figs.

TOOTHACHE
Herbal remedies: Clove oil or finely ground clove powder, banyan-tree sap, honey, onion juice, cashew leaves, coconut oil, asafoetida, fresh mango flowers, burnt mango leaves, nutmeg, mustard oil, sesame-seed oil, green cardamom seeds, dried ginger and liquorice.

CAVITIES IN THE TEETH/CARIES
Herbal remedies: Finely powdered black pepper and cloves.

HYPERACIDITY AND HEARTBURN
Herbal remedies: Indian gooseberry (dried), *terminalia chebula, bael* leaves, liquorice root, banana-tree root, ripe mashed banana, milk, psyllium husk, fresh orange juice, rock salt, buttermilk, fresh ginger juice, honey, omum, coriander and cummin seeds.

INDIGESTION / DYSPEPSIA / BILIOUSNESS
Herbal remedies: Plenty of greens, lime juice, pomegranate rind, cloves, black pepper, cummin seeds, turmeric, rock salt, fenugreek seeds, buttermilk, fresh ginger, mint, fennel, fresh pineapple or pomegranate juice, holy basil-leaf juice, dried ginger powder, jaggery, milk, roasted wheat, broken-wheat porridge, banana, neem juice, neem leaves, cooked rice, long pepper seeds, holy basil juice, *bael* fruit, tamarind pulp and yoghurt.

CONSTIPATION
Herbal remedies: Salads, green vegetables, honey, fresh lime juice, pulp of a ripe *bael* fruit, jaggery, tamarind water, ground peppercorns, asafoetida, omum, cummin and curry-leaf chutney (with black pepper and dried ginger powder) with rice and hot ghee, fresh onion shoots, *terminalia chebula,* liquorice, fennel, Indian gooseberry, spinach, beetroot leaves, fenugreek leaves, green onion stalks, apples, ripe bananas, papayas, oranges, ripe mangoes, grapes, pears, figs, almonds, castor oil and china grass.

BELCHING / FLATULENCE
Herbal remedies: Bicarbonate of soda, fresh lime juice, fresh ginger juice, dried ginger powder, garlic, turmeric, rock salt, *omum,* fenugreek seeds, cloves, bay leaves, orange peel, green cardamom, fennel, mint leaves, betel (leaf), cardamom, rose jelly, catechu and quicklime, asafoetida, tamarind, lightly roasted cummin seeds.

COLIC / CRAMPS IN THE ABDOMEN
Herbal remedies: Lime juice, ginger juice, rock salt, tamarind-leaf paste, omum, ripe bael-fruit pulp, jaggery and radish juice.

DIARRHOEA
Herbal remedies: Apple, a glass of boiled water with a pinch of salt and a level teaspoon of sugar, unripe *bael* fruit, cummin seeds, cinnamon, dry ginger, honey, fresh coriander leaves, green cardamom powder, powdered fig-tree bark, buttermilk, fennel powder, dried mango-flower powder, the kernels of jambul and mango seeds, the pounded bark of the jambul tree, tender jambul leaves or leaf buds, water chestnuts, the dried and powdered bark of the banyan tree, nutmeg, unripe banana, ghee, cloves, coriander seeds, yoghurt, tamarind pulp, banana-flower juice, fresh mint-leaf juice, lime juice, fresh drumstick-leaf juice, pomegranate juice, bottle-gourd juice, carrot soup, pounded peepul-tree bark, rose petals and fenugreek seeds.

DYSENTERY
Herbal remedies: All the remedies for diarrhoea, as well as dried coriander seeds, buttermilk, ripe *bael* fruit, jaggery, ginger juice, fresh lime juice, dried orange peel, seeds of the black grape, mango and pomegranate flowers, fenugreek seeds, yoghurt,

fenugreek leaves, black raisins, dry ginger powder, hot milk, castor oil and psyllium-husk powder.

JAUNDICE / HEPATITIS
Herbal remedies: Sugar cane and sugar cane juice, lime juice, radish-leaf juice, snake-gourd leaf, coriander seeds, split red gram leaves, *bael* leaves, buttermilk, tender papaya leaves, turmeric, yoghurt, banana, Indian gooseberry, jaggery, mint juice, ginger, honey and *phyllanthus amarus*.

GALLSTONES
Herbal remedies: Artichokes, beetroots and beetroot juice, carrot juice and pears.

INTESTINAL WORMS
Herbal remedies (for adults): Crushed cloves of garlic, milk, neem flowers, ghee, dried neem-leaf powder, powdered neem-tree bark, powdered and dried mango-seed kernel, buttermilk, bitter-gourd seeds, bittergourd juice, the dried roots of the banana plant, pomegranate-root bark, honey, cloves, fenugreek seeds, dried Indian gooseberries, flame of the forest-flower seeds, drumsticks, pumpkin seeds, walnuts, fresh cabbage juice, dried papaya seeds, unripe papaya juice, castor oil, lime juice, papaya leaves and powdered betel nut.

Herbal remedies (for children): Fresh neem flowers, tender green neem leaves, omum, black peppers, grated ginger, fennel, jaggery, rice, edible oil, radish juice, rock salt, dried pulp of the aloe leaf, apple juice, cane-sugar or molasses vinegar, chickpeas, carrot juice, coconut paste, castor oil and hot milk.

RENAL STONES
Herbal remedies: Holy basil, honey, celery, figs, white radish, banana stem, horse gram, linseed, lime juice, parsley, barley, melon root and seeds.

DIABETES
Herbal remedies: Jambul-seed powder, milk, turmeric powder, jambul-tree bark, fenugreek needs, Indian gooseberry powder and juice, honey, lime juice, bitter gourd juice and powder, bitter gourd-leaf juice, asafoetida, black gram dal, sandalwood paste curry, leaves, tender mango and neem leaves, dried mango buds or dried mango flowers, cummin seed powder, fresh cabbage juice, dry ginger powder, dried fennel powder, figs and fig-seed powder, and dried bark of the banyan tree.

ARTHRITIS
Herbal remedies: Beetroot and beetroot juice, beetroot leaves, fresh pineapple juice, apple-cider vinegar, honey, celery and celery juice, carrot juice, cucumber juice, spinach juice, asparagus and asparagus seeds, fenugreek seeds, omum, black cummin seeds, raw potato juice, bitter gourd juice, wheatgrass or sprouted wheatgerm, tender green Bengal gram, garlic, sesame seeds, fenugreek leaves, liquorice root, dried ginger powder, cummin powder, black-pepper powder, Indian gooseberry, *terminalia chebula, terminalia belerica,* castor oil, milk and powdered green cardamom.

Massages and local applications: Castor leaves, castor oil, pounded castor seeds, pounded mustard seeds, mustard oil, banyan leaves, garlic, sesame-seed oil, kerosene oil, aloe-leaf pulp, onion juice, warmed onion-bulb mash, neem oil and *omum*.

BACKACHE
Herbal remedies: Foods high in vitamin-C, for example, cabbage, guava, kivi, papaya and Indian gooseberry. All the remedies for arthritis will help in alleviating backache.

MUSCLE STRAINS / SPRAINS / TENDONITIS
Herbal remedies: Sesame-seed oil, sunflower oil, turpentine, kerosene, camphor, sunflower oil, garlic, oil, mustard oil, ginger paste, turmeric powder, eucalyptus leaves, mint leaves, cloves, coriander leaves and coconut oil.

CHILBLAINS
Herbal remedies: Peppercorns, mustard or sesame-seed oil, honey, glycerine, egg white, wholemeal flour, any edible vegetable oil, lime juice, marigold

flowers, spring onions, leeks, onion juice, garlic juice, hot mashed potato paste and warm oatmeal porridge.

BLISTERS
Herbal remedies: Fresh aloe leaf, garlic juice, olive oil and fresh spring-onion juice.

CHAPPED LIPS AND DRY SKIN
Herbal remedies: Any edible vegetable oil, ghee, butter, oatmeal, gram flour, yoghurt, fresh milk cream, turmeric, powdered lentils, glycerine, rose water and lime juice.

FUNGAL SKIN INFECTIONS
Herbal remedies: Black Bengal gram, honey, ground tamarind seeds, lime juice, fresh henna-leaf paste, turmeric powder, sesame-seed oil, fresh turmeric, holy basil-leaf paste and juice, mustard-seed paste, flame of the forest flower seeds, dried and powdered bark of the drumstick root, neem leaves, fresh mint juice, ground and dried papaya seeds, unripe papaya slices and *terminalia chebula.*

FRECKLES / BLEMISHES / SPOTS
Herbal remedies: Lentils, lime juice, honey, salt, orange peel, rose water, jambul seeds, dried pumpkin-seed paste, olive oil, almonds, milk, gram flower, yoghurt, turmeric, buttermilk and sesame-seed oil.

ACNE
Herbal remedies: Buttermilk, jambul-seed paste, gram flower, lentil powder, turmeric powder, roasted and ground mustard seeds, dried and powdered orange peel, *buchanania latifolia,* nutmeg powder, sandalwood powder, black pepper powder, holy basil-leaf juice, neem-leaf juice, milk, camphor powder, ghee, puréed tomatoes, oatmeal, honey, Fuller's earth, fresh potato juice, garlic paste, dried and ground onion seeds, lime juice, yoghurt, neem-leaf or lime-leaf paste, finely ground cinnamon, fenugreek seed and fenugreek-leaf paste.

BLACKHEADS
Herbal remedies: Dried orange peel, tomato purée, onion-seed paste, yoghurt, lentil paste and ripe papaya pulp.

ALLERGIC RASHES / URTICARIA
Herbal remedies: Powdered rock salt, bicarbonate of soda, ginger juice, honey, mint juice and sandalwood paste.

ECZEMA
Herbal remedies: Freshly-made ghee, dried peel of watermelon, melon, diluted neem decoction, neem leaves, turmeric powder or fresh turmeric root, sesame-seed oil, bark of the mango and acacia trees, decoction made of the bark of the peepul tree, sandalwood paste, nutmeg paste, camphor powder and plenty of green vegetables and fruit.

VARICOSE VEIN ULCERS
Herbal remedies: An infusion of marigold flowers, sage, geranium, neem leaves or holy-basil leaves.

HAIR PROBLEMS
Herbal remedies: Fresh neem leaves, soap-nut decoction, coconut oil, Chinese hibiscus, curry leaves, lime peel, fenugreek seeds and paste, mung dal and almond oil.

WOUNDS
Herbal remedies: Fresh garlic juice, garlic paste, aloe-leaf juice, neem-leaf paste, turmeric, papaya-leaf paste, liquorice powder, honey, ghee, ripe bittergourd paste, sugar, and a betel leaf or thin banana leaf.

BITES AND STINGS
Herbal remedies: For ant bites and bee, wasp or hornet stings, salt, paste of bicarbonate of soda and water, parsley juice and honey.

MINOR BURNS
Herbal remedies: Ripe banana pulp, henna-leaf or pomegranate-leaf paste, potato juice, honey, tender

banyan-tree leaves, tender *zizyphus jujuba* leaves, clove powder honey, bicarbonate of soda, buttermilk, yoghurt, beaten egg white and ground chalk paste mixed with linseed oil.

CORNS / CALLUSES / ROUGH HEELS
Herbal remedies: Soap-nut solution, coconut oil, sesame-seed oil, olive oil, castor oil, fresh butter, ghee, shredded lemon peel, uncooked tomatoes and fresh pineapple.

DOG BITE
Herbal remedies: Red chilli powder / paste, asafoetida powder, onion juice and honey.

LEECHES
Herbal remedies: A pinch of salt.

SNAKE BITE
Herbal remedies: Lavender leaves, powdered alum, ghee, the bark of the flame of the forest tree and ginger.

POISONING
Herbal remedies: Tea with charcoal, milk with charcoal, milk, beaten egg whites, a weak starch solution, e.g., cooked rice water or a thin flour solution.

STRESS-RELATED DISORDERS
Herbal remedies: Massages with herbs such as holy basil, fennel, geranium, thyme and marigold; soothing herbal teas made with holy basil, mint, nutmeg, cinnamon, fenugreek seeds, fennel and lemon; also lime juice, honey, orange juice, plenty of greens, salads, vegetables and fruits.

SEXUAL DEBILITY AND WEAKNESS
Herbal remedies: Hot milk, peppercorns, honey, long pepper, almonds, turmeric, saffron, onion seeds, onions—cooked or uncooked—garlic, ghee, asafoetida, banyan-tree sap, dry hibiscus-flower powder, nutmeg powder, a half-boiled egg, wheat, poppy seeds, fenugreek seeds, fresh Indian gooseberry juice, pomegranate-seed powder, sesame seeds, jaggery, omum, kernel of tamarind seeds, drumstick leaves and seeds, and asparagus root

PERIOD PAINS
Herbal remedies: Herbal teas with ginger, honey or sugar, sesame seeds, fennel, aloe-vera leaf; also ripe papaya, carrot juice and parsley soup.

VAGINAL DISCHARGE / IRRITATION
Herbal remedies: Aloe-leaf juice, honey, asparagus juice, hibiscus-flower paste, henna-leaf juice, saffron, milk, dried and pounded bark of the fig and banyan trees, dried pomegranate rind, peepul-tree bark, buttermilk, Indian gooseberry juice and paste, ripe banana, cooked banana flowers or banana-flower juice, palm candy, dried Indian gooseberry-root powder, yoghurt and apple-cider vinegar.

MORNING SICKNESS
Herbal remedies: Powdered green cardamom seeds, honey, roasted gram, orange juice, orange rind, ginger, lime juice, pepper, chillies, cinnamon, onion, lime-peel pickles, tamarind, unripe mango and cloves.

Glossary

ENGLISH NAME	BOTANICAL NAME	HINDI NAME
—	*Acacia concuine*	Shikakai
—	*Buchanania latifolia*	Charoli
—	*Calotropis gigantea*	Arkh
—	*Grewia Asiatica*	Phalsa
—	*Momordica cochinchinensis*	Kheksa
—	*Phyllanthus amarus*	Bhui amla
—	*Psyllium*	Isabgol
—	*Terminalia belerica*	Behera
—	*Terminalia chebula*	Harad
Acacia	*Acacia senegal*	Babul
	Achras sapota	Chiku
Aloe	*Aloe vera*	Ghrita kumari
Amaranth stem	*Amaranthus gangeticus*	Cholai ki dandi
Areca nut	*Areca catechu*	Supari
Arusa	*Justica adhatoda*	Simha mukhi
Asafoetida	*Ferula foetida*	Hing
Ash gourd	*Benincasa hispida*	Petha
Bael fruit	*Aegle marmelos*	Bael
Banana	*Musa sapientum*	Kela
Banyan tree	*Ficus benghalensis*	Burgad
Barberry	*Berberis aristata*	Rasaunt
Bengal gram	*Cicer arietinum*	Chana dal
Bermuda grass	*Cynodon dactylon*	Durva grass
Betel	*Piper betel*	Paan ka patta
Bitter gourd	*Momordica charantia*	Karela
Black cummin	*Nigella sativa*	Shahi jeera
Black gram	*Phaseolus mungo roxb*	Urad dal
Bottle gourd	*Lagenaria vulgaris*	Lauki
Brazilian mimosa	*Mimosa humilis*	Lajwanti
Brinjal	*Solanum melongena*	Baingan
Cashewnut	*Anacardium occidentale*	Kaju
Castor	*Ricinus communis*	—
Catechu	*Acacia catechu*	Katha
Chillies	*Capsicum annum*	Mirch
Chiretta	*Swertia chireta*	Chiraita
Cluster beans	*Cyamopsis tetragon olaba*	Guar ki phali
Coriander	*Coriandrum sativum*	Dhania
Cucumber	*Cucumis sativus*	Khira

255

English	Botanical name	Hindi
Cummin seeds	Cummin cyminum	Jeera
Curry leaves	Murraya koenigii	Kadhi patta
Custard apple	Annona reticulata	Seetaphal
Drumstick	Moringa oleifera	Saijan
Fennel	Foeniculum vulgare	Saunf
Fenugreek	Trigonella foenum-graecum	Methi
Flame of the forest	Butea frondosa	Palash
Grape	Vitis vinifera	Angoor
Green gram	Phaseolus aureus roxb	Mung dal
Groundnut	Arachis hypogaea	Moongphali
Guava	Psidium guajava	Amrud
Henna	Lawsonia inermis	Mehendi
Holy basil	Ocimum santum	Tulsi
Horse gram	Dolichos biflorus	Kulthi dal
Indian gooseberry	Phyllanthus emblica officinalis	Amla
Jujube	Zizyphus jujuba	Ber
Jambul	Eugenia jambolana	Jamun
Kidney bean	Phaseolus vulgaris	Moth dal
Ladies' fingers / okra	Abelmoschus esculentus	Bhindi
Lentil	Lens esculenta	Masur dal
Lime	Citrus acida	Nimbu
Linseed	Linum usitatissimum	Alsi
Long pepper	Piper longum	Peepali
Lotus stem	Nelumbium nelumbo	Kamal gatta
Maize	Zea mays	Bhutta
Mint	Mentha spicata	Pudina
Neem	Azadirachta Indica	Neem
Night jasmine	Nyctanthes arbortristis	Parijat
Omum	Trachyspermum ammi	Ajwain
Papaya	Carica papaya	Papita
Pistachio	Pistacio vera	Pista
Plantain flower	Musa sapientum	Kela ka phool
Pomegranate	Punica granatum	Anar
Pumpkin	Cucurbita maxima	Kaddu
Red gram (split)	Cajanus cajan	Arahar dal
Ridge gourd	Luffa acutangula	Torai
Safflower seeds	Carthamus tinctorius	Kardi
Sesame seeds	Sesamum orientale	Til
Snake gourd	Trichosanthes angina	Chichinga
Soap nut	---	Reetha
Sunflower seeds	Helianthus annus	Surya mukhi
Tamarind	Tamarindus indica	Imli
Vegetable marrow	Cureurbita pepo	Safed kaddu
Water chestnut	Trapa bispinosa	Singhara
White goosefoot	Chenopodium album	Bathua saag